Kevin S. Seybold is Professor of Psychology at Grove City College, Pennsylvania, USA.

EXPLORATIONS IN NEUROSCIENCE, PSYCHOLOGY AND RELIGION

In the 1990s great strides were taken in clarifying how the brain is involved in behaviors that, in the past, had seldom been studied by neuroscientists or psychologists. This book explores the progress begun during that momentous decade in understanding why we behave, think and feel the way we do, especially in those areas that interface with religion. What is happening in the brain when we have a religious experience? Is the soul a product of the mind which is, in turn, a product of the brain? If so, what are the implications for the Christian belief in an afterlife? If God created humans for the purpose of having a relationship with him, should we expect to find that our spirituality is a biologically evolved human trait? What effect might a disease such as Alzheimer's have on a person's spirituality and relationship with God?

Neuroscience and psychology are providing information relevant to each of these questions, and many Christians are worried that their religious beliefs are being threatened by this research. Kevin Seybold attempts to put their concerns to rest by presenting some of the scientific findings coming from these disciplines in a way that is understandable yet non-threatening to Christian belief.

Ashgate Science and Religion Series

Series Editors

Science and religion have often been thought to be at loggerheads but much contemporary work in this flourishing interdisciplinary field suggests this is far from the case. The *Ashgate Science and Religion Series* presents exciting new work to advance interdisciplinary study, research and debate across key themes in science and religion, exploring the philosophical relations between the physical and social sciences on the one hand and religious belief on the other. Contemporary issues in philosophy and theology are debated, as are prevailing cultural assumptions arising from the 'post-modernist' distaste for many forms of reasoning. The series enables leading international authors from a range of different disciplinary perspectives to apply the insights of the various sciences, theology and philosophy and look at the relations between the different disciplines and the rational connections that can be made between them. These accessible, stimulating new contributions to key topics across science and religion will appeal particularly to individual academics and researchers, graduates, postgraduates and upper-undergraduate students.

Other titles published this series:

Theology and Modern Physics
Peter E. Hodgson
978-0-7546-3622-9 (hbk)
978-0-7546-3623-6 (pbk)

From Human to Posthuman
Christian Theology and Technology in a Postmodern World
Brent Waters
978-0-7546-3914-5 (hbk)
978-0-7546-3915-2 (pbk)

God's Action in Nature's World
Essays in Honour of Robert John Russell
Edited by Ted Peters and Nathan Hallanger
978-0-7546-5556-5 (hbk)

Explorations in Neuroscience, Psychology and Religion

KEVIN S. SEYBOLD
Grove City College, Pennsylvania, USA

ASHGATE

Published by

Ashgate Publishing Limited
Gower House
Croft Road
Aldershot
Hampshire GU11 3HR
England

Ashgate Publishing Company
Suite 420
101 Cherry Street
Burlington, VT 05401-4405
USA

Ashgate website: http://www.ashgate.com

British Library Cataloguing in Publication Data
Seybold, Kevin S.
Explorations in Neuroscience, Psychology and Religion. –
(Ashgate Science and Religion Series)
1. Neurosciences. 2. Neurosciences – Religious aspects – Christianity 3. Neurosciences – Religious aspects.. 4. Psychology and religion. 5. Religion and science.
I. Title
612.8'01

Library of Congress Cataloging-in-Publication Data
Seybold, Kevin S., 1956–
Explorations in Neuroscience, Psychology, and Religion / Kevin S. Seybold.
p. cm. – (Ashgate Science and Religion Series)
Includes bibliographical references and index.
1. Brain – Religious aspects – Christianity. 2. Theological anthropology – Christianity. 3. Psychology and religion. I. Title.
[DNLM: 1. Neuropsychology – methods. 2. Religion and Psychology. 3. Brain – physiology. 4. Christianity – psychology. WL 103.5S519e 2006]
BT702.S49 2007
261.5'15–dc22 2006022470

The book has been printed on acid-free paper.

ISBN 978-0-7546-5563-3

Printed and bound in Great Britain by MPG Books Ltd, Bodmin, Cornwall.

Contents

List of Figures

Acknowledgements

Chaim Potok starts his book *In the Beginning* saying 'All beginnings are hard'. When it comes to writing, I think I agree with him. The idea for this book goes back to the mid 1990s when an explosion of research on the brain occurred, some of that research having direct implications for religious experience, belief and practice. The actual writing of these pages did not begin, however, until several years later with the help of a grant from the John Templeton Foundation to participate in the Oxford Seminars on Science and Christianity sponsored by the Council for Christian Colleges and Universities (CCCU). Over the course of three summers I enjoyed and greatly benefited from the friendship and intellectual inspiration of my fellow participants. Their impact on my life is considerable and will not be forgotten. Many thanks to the Foundation and the CCCU for the opportunity to attend these seminars held at Wycliffe Hall, Oxford University, and to the faculty and staff at Wycliffe. Special appreciation goes to Alister McGrath and John Roche who organized the summer programs. I have also benefited from many colleagues, here at Grove City College and elsewhere, who have influenced (subtly or more directly) my thinking on neuroscience, psychology and religion. In particular, I thank Peter Hill for his sustained support and friendship over many years, and Heather Looy, Kevin Reimer and Brent Waters for their insights and encouragement. I am grateful to Sarah Lloyd, my editor, for her recommendation that this book be considered for the Ashgate Science and Religion Series and others at Ashgate who provided helpful advice in the editorial process. Finally, I thank my son, Adam, for creatively and helpfully challenging my own worldviews and my wife, Ginny, for sharing the last 25 years with me. It is to her that I dedicate this book.

KEVIN SEYBOLD
January 2007

To my wife, Ginny

Introduction

My wife and I had been in the room for about twelve hours. In a bed, near death, lay my mother. At 80 years of age, my mother enjoyed a relatively healthy life, living on her own, driving around town on errands, and occasionally visiting family members in neighboring states. While my sister lived in the same town and certainly helped her when needed, my mother was nevertheless able to live as most elderly prefer, in her own home. In the last five months of her life, however, my mother began to carry a small oxygen tank with her wherever she went. Her condition was officially listed as chronic restrictive lung disease, a problem she had apparently had for years, but one that had recently created a health concern. Now, she was unconscious, breathing irregularly, lying in a nursing home bed. Eventually, my mother took a breath, exhaled, and did not breathe again. What happened to my mother at that instant? Where did the woman who gave me birth, cared for me during my childhood, and never stopped loving or worrying about me 'go' at the moment of her death? Or, did the person who was my mother 'leave' even before her body took its last breath?

A dramatic increase in research on the brain took place during the 1990s, and many of the findings made in neuroscience, psychology and related fields since that time have implications to questions such as those above. Great strides were made in the last fifteen years in elucidating the brain mechanisms involved in a variety of behaviors that, in the past, were seldom, if ever, studied by neuroscientists or psychologists. While most people do not necessarily have an interest in quantum physics, chaos theory or physical chemistry, many are nevertheless interested in behavior, their own and that of others. Not only are people interested in behavior, they tend to form theories of behavior as well. Psychologists use the term 'attribution' to refer to this tendency of people to try to explain their own or other's actions.

This book discusses some of the progress begun during the momentous decade of the 1990s in understanding why we behave the way we do, especially in those areas that interface with religion. The book begins with some of the basics of neuroscience and psychology. What are the origins of these disciplines, what methods do they use, what do they say about behavior, and how do they understand human nature? Religion is then discussed in a similar fashion. What is religion, what is its origin, and how does the specific religion of Christianity view human nature? Following these chapters, the book considers how science is actually practiced today, and discusses how science might be related to religion. This is an important area, not only for Christian scientists, but also for other people of faith who live in a world that is increasingly becoming dependent on the advances made by science (and technology) and influenced by a scientific worldview that is often seen as being too naturalistic and reductionistic.

The second half of the book consists of reviews of the latest developments in neuroscience, psychology and cognitive science written for the 'person in the pew', a person who might read the May, 2001 *Newsweek* cover story 'God and the Brain' or see *The God Gene* in the bookstore and wonder what scientific discovery had been made or be concerned that science is 'once again' overstepping its bounds and challenging or dismissing belief in God. It is in these chapters that I describe the latest findings on a handful of topics that I believe will be of interest to believing Christians. In addition to describing the research, however, I attempt to show how the research relates to the Christian faith. Should a Christian be concerned that certain brain areas show changes in activity level during prayer? What are the implications for the Christian belief in an afterlife of research suggesting that the soul is a product of the mind (which is, in turn, a product of the brain)? What effect might diseases of the brain such as Alzheimer's or Parkinson's have on a person's spirituality and relationship to God? Many Christians are worried that their religious beliefs, beliefs that are precious and important to them, are being steadily challenged and, in the opinion of some, replaced by facts discovered through science. I hope to put these concerns to rest by presenting some of the scientific findings coming from neuroscience and psychology in a way that is understandable yet non-threatening to Christian belief.

It is often said that science and religion are in conflict, and there have been times in history where that has seemed to be the case. In actuality, however, science and religion are not contradictory or in conflict. Throughout history, the typical pattern is one of science and religion complementing each other. Reality is complex and multilayered, and it takes multiple perspectives to develop a complete and accurate picture of that reality. Science and religion (as well as other ways of knowing) are both required, and a Christian needs to be aware of how these two perspectives 'fit together' into an understandable pattern. Believers need not avoid science or fear what science, when practiced honestly, says about nature and who we are. It is possible to be a person of faith and at the same time be well informed about the latest discoveries of science, even those findings coming from neuroscience and psychology that have direct implications to important and cherished religious beliefs. It is in this spirit that the following chapters were written and, hopefully, will be read.

Chapter 1

Neuroscience

The Society for Neuroscience is a professional organization that was formed in 1970 with around 500 charter members. Today the Society has over 36,000 members from around the globe and is the largest group of scientists devoted to studying the brain. At a recent annual meeting in San Diego, California, nearly 31 000 people attended the five-day convention meant to provide a means of disseminating the very latest research results on the brain, the most complicated organ of the body. To go to an annual meeting of the Society for Neuroscience is to be impressed by the size and range of the research that takes place in the neurosciences. Alzheimer's disease, ion channels, memory, long-term potentiation, motor systems, gender, membrane receptors, mood disorders, vision, pain, the immune system, ethics, cell division, neurotransmitters and Schwann cells are just a few of the topics one could read or hear about at the annual meeting. So many researchers present their findings at the convention that only the largest of the convention centers in the United States can hold the throng. A relatively small number of researchers present their work orally in 'paper sessions' attended by a few dozen to a few hundred interested peers. The vast majority of the research is reported in 'poster sessions'. The results of literally thousands of research studies are presented on six-foot by four-foot standing posters that fill the floor of the convention center. Researchers roam from poster to poster to read the latest findings in the areas of investigation that interest them. In addition to the poster and paper presentations, there are more informal and relaxed social gatherings of people interested in similar subjects. Thus, there is the Vision Social, the Cajal Club Social, the Hippocampus Social, the Songbird Social, and the ominous-sounding Cell Death Social, among many others. There really is something for everyone.

Despite its enormous size, the convention is remarkably well run. Transportation is provided from outlying hotels to the convention center, food is easily available at the convention center itself or the many restaurants in the surrounding area, and the program runs from mid-morning to late evening. Attending an annual meeting of the Society for Neuroscience is both mentally stimulating and physically exhausting. It does have, however, a kind of bazaar-like feeling, with people moving from poster to poster or seminar room to seminar room listening to the spiel of the scientists 'hawking' their research results.

A Brief History of Neuroscience

As suggested by the tremendous growth in the Society since its founding, scientific interest in the brain increased significantly in the latter part of the twentieth century.

The number of graduate programs in neuroscience also grew during this same period, as did the number of academic journals devoted to research on the brain. Despite this recent surge in interest in the brain and nervous system, evidence from paleontology suggests that early humans already suspected that damage to the brain could not only produce disabling injuries, but could also lead to death itself (Finger, 1994, p. 3). Trephines, holes drilled in the skull, indicate that humans 10 000 years ago believed the brain was somehow involved in the higher mental functions, in that the trephines were associated with rituals whereby the survivor was seen as having special or perhaps magical mental powers. Another view of the trephines is that the boring of the holes in the skull was a treatment for headaches, mental disorders or perhaps even demon possession (Finger, 1994, p. 5).

In ancient Egypt and Greece, as well as in ancient China, there were differences of opinion as to which organ of the body was the most important in so far as the 'mental' capacities of the individual were concerned. Some believed that the brain was the center for mind or soul, but a significant number of others held that the heart (or perhaps the liver) was the seat of the faculties associated with soul. The Greek philosopher Plato (*c.* 427–347 BC), for example, argued for a three-part soul, one part of which (the vegetative) was associated with the liver, one (the vital) with the heart, and one (the immortal, rational soul) with the head. Plato's student Aristotle (384–322 BC), however, held that while the soul was the form of the body (it was both everywhere and nowhere), the heart was the center of intellectual activity (Marshall and Magoun, 1998, p. 27). This made sense to Aristotle, in that, being an anatomist and embryologist, the heart was the first organ he could see in the embryo (Zimmer, 2004, p. 13). In early Christianity, the heart became the site for the passions as well as for moral conscience (Zimmer, 2004, p. 16). In the famous painting 'Light of the World' by William Holman Hunt which hangs in St Paul's Cathedral in London, it is at the heart's door that Jesus knocks, waiting to be let in.

The Roman doctor Galen (130–*c.* 200) suggested that the liver, heart and brain together are involved in the soul-like powers of the body. The liver filled the blood with natural spirits which were then passed on to the heart, where they were pumped, along with the blood, to the various muscles and organs of the body to be used as nourishment. Some of the blood, however, went from the heart to the head, where the blood passed through a series of vessels called the *rete mirabile* (marvelous network). Passing through this network transformed the natural or vital spirits in the blood into animal spirits which were capable of thought as well as sensation and movement (Zimmer, 2004, p. 15). These animal spirits filled the hollow cavities in the brain called the ventricles, so while the brain was recognized in Galen's scheme, it was actually the ventricles that were crucial. The brain, like the heart, served as a pump; intellectual capacity itself was located in the hollow cavities within the head.

Galen made his observations from the dissection of animals and random encounters with wounded soldiers. (Human dissection was prohibited in the Roman Empire.) Relying on these observations, and despite his reverence for Aristotle's work, Galen identified the importance of the brain over the heart, based upon his tracing of the nerves from the sense organs to the brain. While these dissections were crucial to the development of his theory, the fact that he did not perform dissections on humans resulted in errors and limitations in his theories. For example, the very important role of the *rete mirabile* in the transformation of vital spirits to animal spirits in the brain is diminished when one recognizes that there is no marvelous network in humans (Finger, 2000, p. 47).

Galen's view of the soul was still dominant into the 1600s. During this century, however, the work of Thomas Willis (1621–1675) clarified the importance of the brain itself, not the ventricles, in intellectual and mental functioning. Willis was a physician and experimentalist. Some of his patients experienced various kinds of mental or intellectual disturbances during their lives, and when these patients died, Willis was often able to convince the next of kin to allow him to perform an autopsy or post mortem on the body. As part of this procedure, Willis would remove and dissect the brain in an attempt to correlate the person's intellectual or mental impairment with an observable lesion in brain tissue. As a result of his investigations, Willis increasingly was able to demonstrate that the functions normally attributed to an immaterial soul (located in the heart or brain) were actually performed by the physical structure of the brain itself.

The extent to which these mental and intellectual functions are localizable to specific brain regions became an important area of investigation after Willis and into the twentieth century. (Actually, it remains a controversial topic even today, as we will see in later chapters.) Franz Joseph Gall (1758–1828) believed that the cortex of the brain was composed of several distinct regions, each of which was responsible for a particular mental faculty. For example, there were regions, unique to humans, which controlled wisdom, kindness, religious sentiment, even poetic talent. In addition, there were faculties humans shared with animals such as pride, vanity, sense of place, and affection. In total, there were 27 different faculties of mind in humans, each with a particular region of the cortex responsible for it. The movement known as phrenology was based upon the notion of localization of function and spread throughout Europe and America. Phrenology, a term never used by Gall but popularized by his disciple Johann Spurzheim, proposed that a person's mental and intellectual capabilities could be determined by feeling a person's skull. The skull, the phrenologists incorrectly believed, corresponded to the underlying brain surface. Excesses in a particular brain region would produce a 'bump' on the skull over that brain area. Deficiencies in a mental or intellectual function would produce a depression in the skull over that region. Thus, one could 'read' a person's skull and determine in what mental and intellectual faculties they excelled or were wanting.

Other brain scientists investigated the role of the cortex in movement and sensation. Eduard Hitzig (1838–1907) discovered that electrical stimulation near the front and on the top of a dog's cortex produced movement of the dog's leg, face or neck muscles on the side opposite the stimulation (Finger, 2000, p. 161). David Ferrier (1843–1928) identified areas in the temporal lobe that seemed to be responsible for hearing and smell, and eventually corroborated the finding of another scientist suggesting the importance of the occipital lobe in vision (Finger, 2000, p. 165). These experimentalists, along with many others, were showing that there were indeed specialized areas of the cerebral cortex, even if the more extreme beliefs of the phrenologists were false.

In the 1830s, the cell theory, the notion that all living things are made of individual cells, was accepted (Finger, 2000, p. 201). This theory, however, did not immediately apply to the nervous system itself. With better staining techniques and stronger microscopes, the cell theory was also accepted for the nervous system by the mid-1860s. Camillo Golgi (1843–1926) developed a silver stain which turned approximately 3 percent of the nerve cells silver and black against a lighter yellow background (Finger, 2000, p. 204). This stain permitted a clearer view of the brain cell and its processes. Modifying and improving on Golgi's staining technique, Santiago Ramón y Cajal (1852–1934) showed that the brain consisted of many individual cells, a concept known as the neuron doctrine.

Obviously, there are many other scientists whose work contributed to the development of contemporary neuroscience, and anything approaching a complete and detailed history of the discipline cannot be attempted in this chapter. This chapter will, however, provide some of the essential principles of neuroscience so that a better understanding of its methods, assumptions and findings will be possible. One of the significant questions occupying philosophy for centuries is that of the relationship between the mind and the body. Today, that question is usually put in the form of: 'What is the relationship between the mind and the brain?' Neuroscientists typically respond to that question by taking a position of monism, which is the view that what we call the mind is actually the brain in action. There are variations of this monist position. There is a completely reductive monism which says that there is nothing but the brain (the mind is simply eliminated from all discussion and consideration). There is also a softer kind of monism which suggests that what we call the mind is a property that emerges from the physical brain. Either way, the material brain is clearly the focus of study in the neurosciences, and the goal is to understand behavior and mental functioning in terms of activity of the nervous system.

Another position taken by neuroscientists is that of naturalism. This view holds that explanations for phenomena, in this case the neural basis of behavior, are to be found in natural processes and mechanisms. Supernatural explanations are to be avoided because the methods of neuroscience, like the methods of other sciences, are only appropriate in the search for natural mechanisms. This is not to say that other, non-natural mechanisms are not possible; it is simply to state that if they exist, science is unable to uncover and detect them. As such, a reductionism in method is followed in the neurosciences. The way to uncover the natural mechanisms underlying the neural basis of behavior is to reduce the complex phenomena to simpler, more manageable pieces. By studying these simpler components, and discovering the natural mechanisms that govern them, one can then begin to put the components together to get an idea of how the larger, more complex whole works. This is the methodology followed, and this methodological reductionism needs to be clearly separated and distinguished from ontological reductionism, which is a philosophical position holding that all of reality can ultimately be reduced to the fundamental principles of chemistry and physics. Methodological reductionism is a way of looking for natural mechanisms underlying some phenomenon. It is not a philosophical position suggesting these underlying natural mechanisms are all that exist of the phenomenon. This view does suggest, however, that science is limited, and is only able to investigate and search for these natural systems.

Basics of Neuroscience: The Neuron

The human nervous system is divided into two basic components: the central and the peripheral nervous systems. The central nervous system (CNS) consists of the brain and spinal cord; the peripheral nervous system (PNS) consists of all neural structures outside of the brain and spinal cord. As mentioned above, the nervous system (both CNS and PNS) consists of individual cells. These cells of the nervous system are called neurons, and neurons are like other cells of the body in many ways. Like other cells (skin, liver, pancreas, and so on) neurons have a cell membrane which defines the cell and keeps some things in the cell and other things out. Neurons also have a cell nucleus which contains genetic information, mitochondria which produce energy for the cell, and many other structures that provide for the basic maintenance of the cell. While neurons share these structures and characteristics with other bodily cells, there is one way in which these neural cells are unlike any other cell in the body. Neurons generate and conduct electrical impulses, and these impulses make up the kind of information that the nervous system processes. Everything we perceive, feel, do and think is made possible through the processing of electrical messages generated by and carried along these cells of the brain, spinal cord and peripheral nervous system.

Neurons come in various shapes and sizes. Some are microscopic in length; others can reach a length of several feet. Despite the variations in their size and shape, all neurons have four principal structures: a soma, dendrites, an axon and several terminal buttons (see Figure 1.1). The *soma* (or cell body) of a neuron contains the nucleus and many of the structures the neuron shares with other cells of the body. The *dendrites* are those parts of the neuron that typically receive information from other neural cells. (On average, a given neuron in the brain will receive this information from around 10 000 other neurons.) The *axon* of the neuron is a singular tube-like process that carries information from the soma of the neuron to the *terminal buttons*, which send the information to other neurons. (On average, a given neuron in the brain will send information to around 10 000 other neurons.) It is estimated that there are between 100 billion and 1000 billion neurons in the human nervous system (Carlson, 2007, p. 30), and some scientists speculate that the number of possible ways these neurons can be interconnected exceeds the number of atoms in the universe. (It is the complexity of the interconnections among neurons that gives the brain its processing power and that results in the emergence of mental states such as consciousness.) The point at which neurons 'interconnect' is called a *synapse*, and this junction between neurons is usually between the terminal button of one neuron and the dendrite of the next. While the term 'junction' suggests actual contact between the neurons, in fact they do not touch. There is a small gap, called the *synaptic cleft*, which separates the two neurons, and this cleft, as discussed below, is an important feature in how these neural cells communicate with each other.

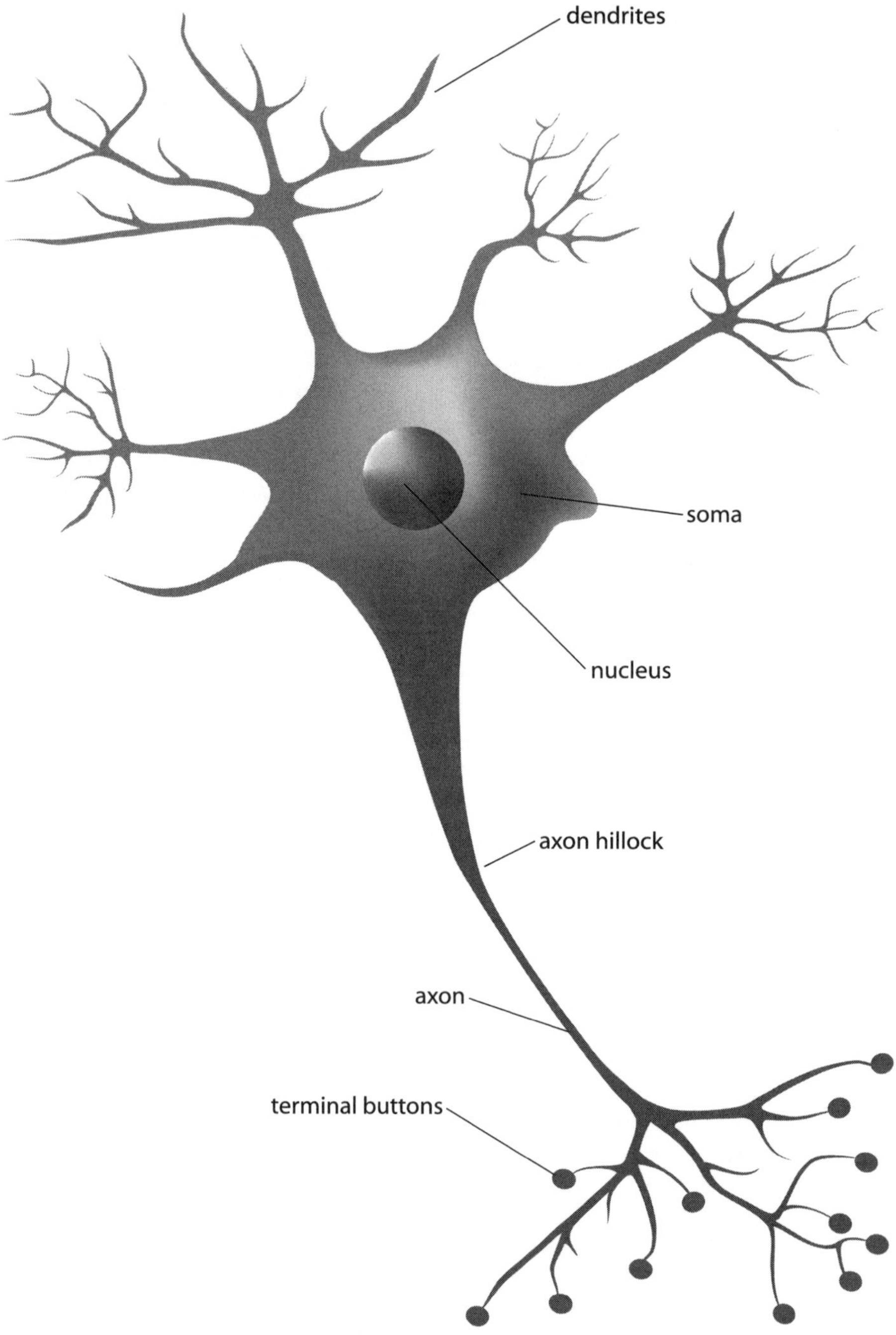

Figure 1.1 The neuron and its principal structures.

Neurons do not exist in isolation, they group together. Within the CNS, a group of somas or cell bodies that are located together is called a *nucleus* (plural nuclei). A bundle or group of axons that are traveling together from one location to another within the CNS is called a *tract*. Within the PNS, a group of cell bodies is called a *ganglion* (plural ganglia), and a bundle of axons is called a *nerve*. Information traveling toward the CNS (or from a lower area to a higher area within the CNS) is called afferent information, and information traveling out of the CNS (or from a higher to a lower area within the CNS) is termed efferent information. So an afferent nerve is carrying electrical impulses toward the brain or spinal cord, and an efferent nerve is carrying electrical impulses away from the brain and spinal cord. An afferent tract is carrying electrical impulses from a lower brain region (for example, the medulla) to a higher brain region (for example, the thalamus), and an efferent tract is carrying these impulses in the opposite direction.

Additional important vocabulary includes directional terms such as anterior (toward the head), posterior (toward the tail), dorsal (toward the top or back), ventral (toward the bottom or front), and medial and lateral (toward the middle and side respectively).

Neurophysiology and the Electrical Impulse

The only kind of information the nervous system can process and understand is in the form of electrical impulses, and these electrical messages are generated within the neuron as a result of the movement of charged molecules through the cell's membrane. Some of these molecules, or ions, have a positive charge, others have a negative charge. The most important of these ions are sodium (Na^+), chloride (Cl^-), potassium (K^+) and a group of negatively charged ions given the label A^-. The membrane of the neuron is semi-permeable, some of ions can pass through, others cannot. In its unexcited state (that is, the neuron is not generating any electrical impulses), the neuron has a relatively large amount of K^+ and A^- ions, and small amounts of Cl^- and Na^+ inside the cell. Outside the cell, there are relatively large amounts of Na^+ and Cl^-, and small amounts of K^+ (A^- is only located inside the cell, as these molecules are too big to pass through the semi-permeable neuron membrane.) The distribution of these ions inside and outside of the neuron creates an electrical potential across the cell membrane, known as the resting potential, and is measured at around -65 mV. (The voltage value is preceded by a negative sign because the inside of the cell is negatively charged in comparison to the outside, and by convention the voltage is based upon the charge inside the neuron.) The distribution of the ions is a function of two forces that are present: the force of diffusion and the electrostatic force. Diffusion tends to force the movement of molecules from regions of higher concentrations to areas of lower concentration. As a result, diffusion would tend to push Na^+ into the cell and K^+ outside of the cell because of the relative distributions of these two ions. The second force that is at work is electrostatic pressure, which is the attractive force between molecules with different signs or the repulsive force of molecules with similar signs. Electrostatic pressure tends to force Na^+ inside the cell because the inside is negatively charged relative to the outside and Na^+ is a positively charged ion. The same pressure tends to keep K^+ inside the cell, because the positively charged potassium is attracted to the negativity inside the neuron. The balance of these two forces maintains the distribution of ions inside and outside the neuron and creates the membrane potential.

When the membrane of the neuron is stimulated, its permeability changes and ion channels, pathways through the membrane, open which allow Na^+ to enter the cell, forced in via electrostatic pressure and by diffusion. As positively charged sodium enters the neuron, it becomes less negative inside, a process called depolarization. (Making the inside of the neuron more negative, hyperpolarization, is also possible, but we will not discuss that process here because it does not lead to the generation of an electrical message.) The membrane potential changes from approximately -65 mV to -64 mV or -63 mV or -62 mV, depending on how much Na^+ enters through the ion channels. If enough Na^+ enters to depolarize the membrane to around -60 mV, the threshold of excitation is reached, all ion channels for sodium open, and there is a massive influx of Na^+ ions into the neuron. As a result of this influx of positively charged sodium ions, the inside of the neuron becomes positively charged *vis-à-vis* the outside. While this reversal of the membrane potential is occurring, potassium channels open and K^+ ions rush out of the cell, forced out due to the combined forces of diffusion and electrostatic pressure. (Not only is there the force of diffusion at work – there is relatively little potassium outside the cell compared to inside the cell – but electrostatic pressure now forces K^+ outside, because the inside of the neuron is now positively charged compared to the outside.) As positively charged K^+ leaves the neuron, the inside becomes less and less positive, eventually returning to its resting potential of -65 mV. This rapid and temporary reversal of the membrane potential (going from -65 mV to around +40 mV and back to -65 mV in about 3 msec) is termed an action potential, and it is this action potential that is the electrical message processed by the nervous system. Everything we see, hear, touch, feel, think and so on is represented in the form of this kind of electrical impulse. All of our behavior is made possible because of the generation of these action potentials within the neurons of the central and peripheral nervous systems. The kind of information processed by the nervous system is electrical in nature.

Neural Communication

In order for these electrical messages to travel from one part of the nervous system to another, neurons must communicate with each other. This process of neural communication occurs at the synapse, the functional connection between the terminal buttons of one neuron and the dendrites (typically) of another neuron (see Figure 1.2). The electrical impulses described above are generated at the part of the neuron where the soma and axon join, a point called the axon hillock. Once this action potential is generated, it is carried down the axon toward the terminal buttons. The arrival of the electrical impulse at the terminal buttons causes the buttons to release a chemical called a neurotransmitter. (Because the electrical impulse cannot 'jump' across the synaptic cleft between the terminal buttons and the dendrites of the next neuron, the electrical message must be temporarily changed into a chemical one.)

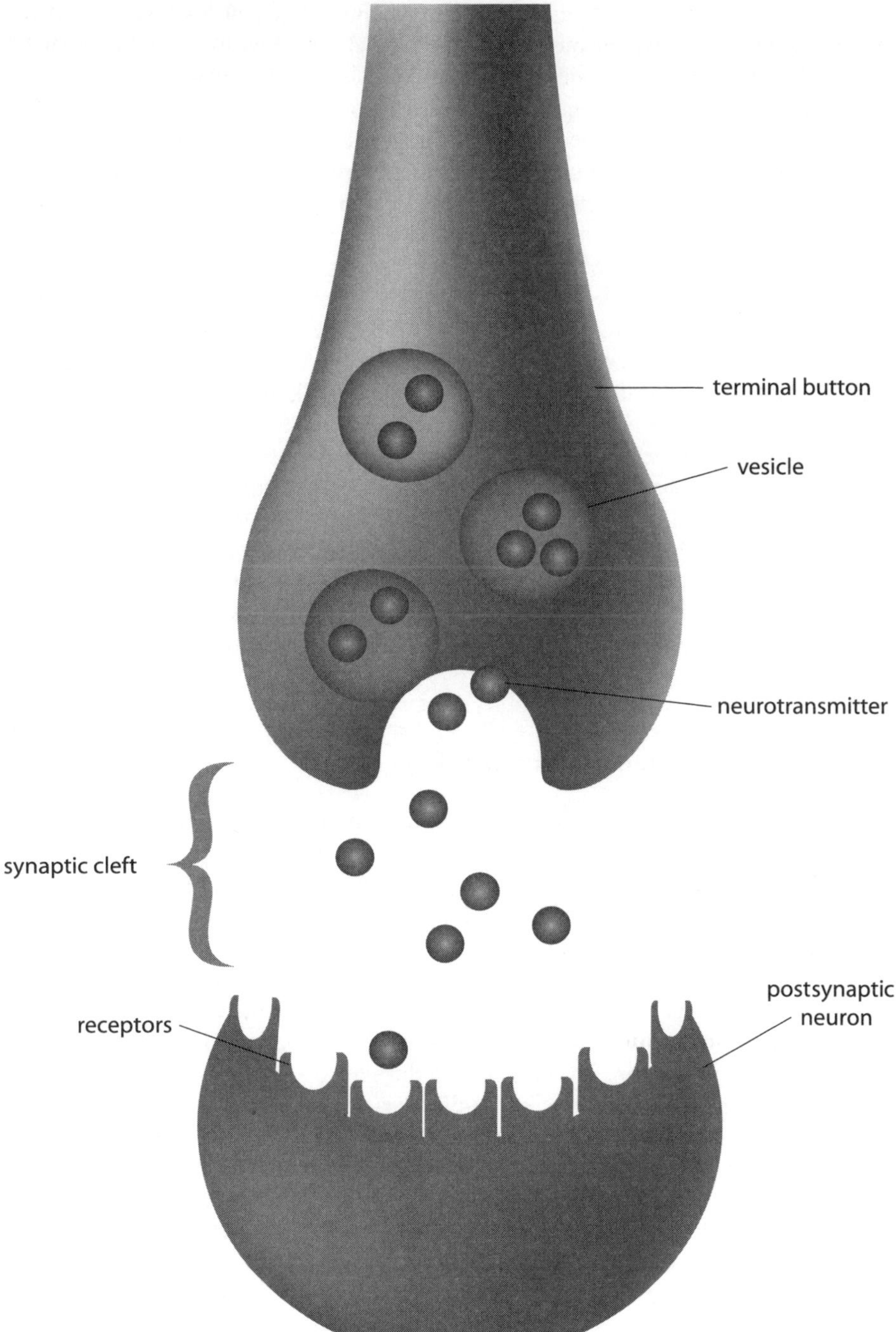

Figure 1.2 The synapse.

The neurotransmitter travels across the synaptic cleft and fits into specialized slots (called receptors) in the membrane of the dendrites of the next, or postsynaptic, neuron. When the neurotransmitter fits into the receptor, the membrane potential at that portion of the receiving neuron is changed (depolarized). If enough depolarization of the postsynaptic neuron occurs, it will generate an action potential at its axon hillock, and the electrical impulse will be sent down the axon to the terminal buttons. Through this process of electrical messages (action potentials) being changed into chemical messages (neurotransmitters) generating new action potentials, information is moved from one part of the nervous system to another.

Each of these neurotransmitters has a slightly different effect on the postsynaptic receptor. To complicate matters even more, there are different receptor types for each of these neurotransmitters, so the effect of the neurotransmitter on the receiving neuron is not always (or usually) as simple as I have described above. Nevertheless, the basic process of one neuron communicating with another is fundamentally as has been described, and is crucial in understanding how the nervous system is involved in controlling our behavior, thinking, feeling and so on. Drugs that affect the brain, the psychoactive drugs, are numerous and have their influence at the synapse and on the exchange of information between neurons. For example, psychoactive drugs can have their effect by increasing or decreasing the release of the neurotransmitter, preventing the synthesis of the neurotransmitter itself, or directly stimulating or blocking the postsynaptic receptor, thereby mimicking or inhibiting the effect of the neurotransmitter.

Organization of the Human Nervous System

The nervous system begins embryologically as a hollow tube on the top service of the embryo (beginning approximately 21 days after conception). This neural tube will continue to develop and give rise to the brain and spinal cord, which make up the central nervous system (CNS). Looking first at the spinal cord, we see that its major function is to send motor information from the brain to the muscles and glands of the body and to carry sensory information from these same bodily structures into the brain. Approximately 44 cm in length and 1 cm in diameter, the spinal cord is divided into distinct sensory or motor pathways, and is protected by the vertebra as well as by a tough covering of tissue called dura mater. Sensory information enters and motor information exits the spinal cord via spinal nerves which make up the peripheral nervous system (see below).

The second part of the CNS is the brain, which weighs about 1400 grams (approximately 3 lb) and consists of hundreds of billions of brain cells. During the course of embryological development, the neural tube grows and differentiates into the major structures of the brain (see Figures 1.3 and 1.4). A few of these principal structures are the medulla, the cerebellum, the thalamus and hypothalamus, the amygdala, the hippocampus and the cerebral cortex. The medulla is considered a brain stem structure, that is to say it is located near where the brain and the spinal cord merge. Cell bodies or nuclei in the medulla control basic life functions such as respiration and regulation of the cardiovascular system. Another structure near the rear portion of the brain is the cerebellum. One of the functions of this structure is to coordinate movement; damage to the cerebellum can result in uncoordinated and jerky movements. The cerebellum is also involved in some kinds of learning, specifically the kind of learning known as classical or Pavlovian conditioning. Certain nuclei in the cerebellum are necessary for classical conditioning to occur. When these cells are damaged, this type of learning is abolished.

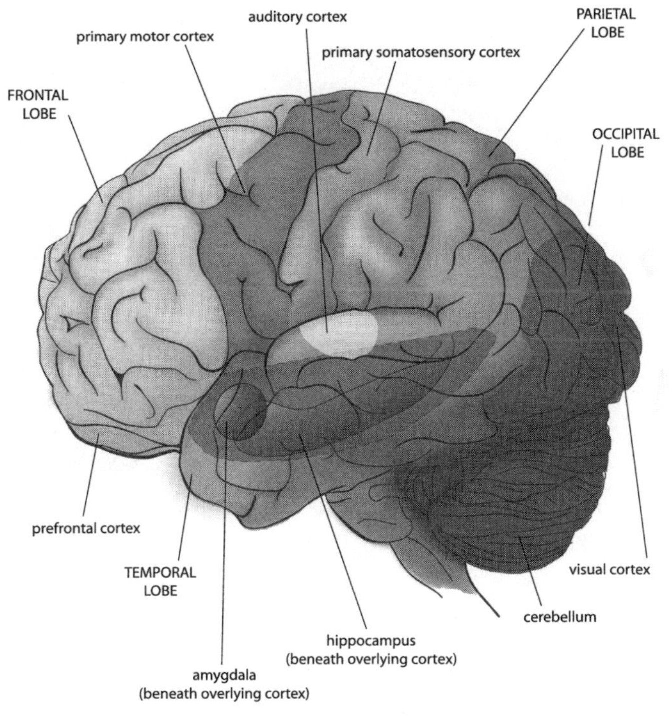

Figure 1.3 A lateral view of the brain.

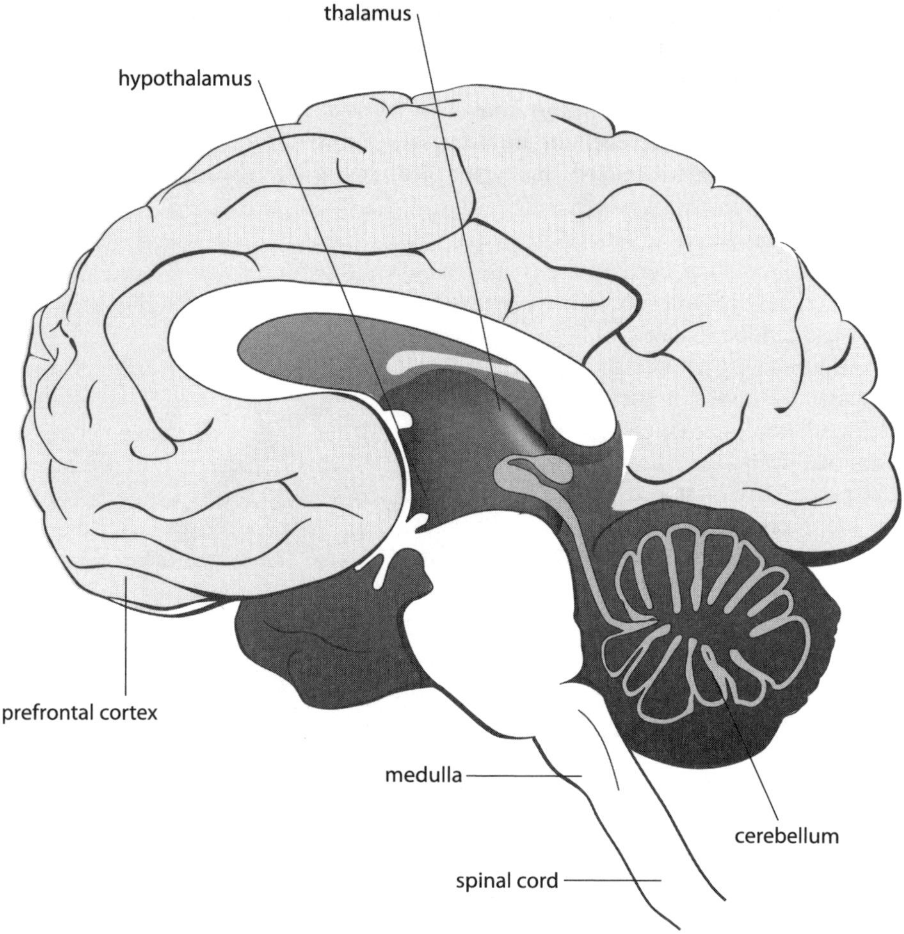

Figure 1.4 A medial view of the brain (left hemisphere removed).

Moving toward the front of the brain (in an anterior direction), the next principal structure to mention is the thalamus. Located more or less in the center of the brain, the thalamus serves as a kind of relay station for many of the senses. A great amount of visual information passes through the thalamus before it is sent on to other brain areas for additional processing. The same is true for auditory information as well as for taste and some touch information. Indeed, much of the information that eventually reaches the cerebral cortex first passes through the thalamus. Situated just below or ventral to the thalamus is the hypothalamus, which contains nuclei that are involved in the survival of the species (for example, eating, fighting, sexual behavior, thermoregulation and so on). In addition, the hypothalamus is attached to and controls the pituitary gland, which is the master gland of the body. Impulses or chemical messages from the hypothalamus travel to the pituitary gland, which stimulates this gland to release hormones that target other glands such as the thyroid, adrenal and gonads, causing these glands to release their particular hormones. For example, in response to a stressor the hypothalamus will release a chemical called corticotrophin-releasing hormone (CRH), which travels to the pituitary gland, causing it to release adrenocorticotropic hormone (ACTH). ACTH in turn travels throughout the body, but has a specific effect on the adrenal cortex lying adjacent to the kidney. At the adrenal cortex, ACTH causes the adrenal gland to release glucocorticoids (for example, cortisol), which helps prepare the body to respond to the stressor experienced in the environment. When the system is functioning properly, the higher levels of circulating cortisol are detected by the hypothalamus, which causes an inhibition of CRH and subsequent suppression of ACTH from the pituitary gland. In this way, a proper balance of hormones is maintained in the body.

Additional structures in the brain are the amygdala and hippocampus. Both are part of a collection of structures called the limbic system, an area involved in the regulation of emotion. The amygdala in particular is implicated in a variety of emotional responses, most notably fear. The hippocampus is also part of this circuit that processes emotion, but it is also involved in learning and memory. Without the hippocampus, no new long-term memories are formed. People with damage to the hippocampus will typically be able to remember the past if those memories were created before the hippocampal damage, but they will not be able to form new declarative memories, memories for events that happened to them or factual information they have recently learned. The hippocampus is also implicated in a number of neurological disorders such as Alzheimer 's disease and schizophrenia.

The most obvious area of the brain when one examines it is the cerebral cortex, the outer few millimeters of surface tissue that surround the brain. The cerebral cortex is distinguished by the many grooves and bumps that are readily apparent. The grooves are called sulci, and the bumps on the surface of the brain are called gyri. Particular sulci divide the surface of the cerebral cortex into four distinct lobes, the frontal, parietal, occipital and temporal lobes. Particular features of these lobes include the primary visual processing center in the occipital lobe at the very posterior portion of the brain. This is the area where some of the earliest processing of visual information occurs. From here, the visual information is sent to adjacent regions of the cortex for additional processing and interpretation.

The temporal lobe contains the primary auditory processing region. As in the visual system, this particular region performs an early analysis of auditory information and forwards its output to other auditory centers for deeper processing. Some language areas are also found here in the temporal lobe, adjacent to the primary auditory cortex. In the parietal lobe is an area of cortex devoted to the processing of somatosensory (touch, temperature, pressure and so on) information from the body. As will be discussed in Chapter 6, other regions of the parietal lobe are thought to be implicated in creating a boundary for the self, a distinction between what is and what is not the self.

The frontal lobe is thought to contain areas responsible for many of the brain functions that are most likely unique to humans. For example, one area called the prefrontal cortex at the very front pole of the brain is implicated in decision making, moral judgments and the development of a theory of mind, the ability to understand or 'read' others' mental states and intentions.

The brain and spinal cord communicate to the rest of the body via the PNS, which consists of 31 pairs of spinal nerves and 12 pairs of cranial nerves. The spinal nerves enter and leave the spinal cord at various locations along its length, and carry motor and sensory information for muscles and glands as well as information from the sensory receptors located throughout the body. The cranial nerves have a similar function, except that they leave the CNS from the ventral surface of the brain and serve primarily the motor and sensory functions of the neck and head. The PNS can be divided into various branches or sub-systems. For example, the first major division of the PNS is into either somatic or autonomic subsystems. The somatic nervous system serves sensory and motor functions for the skeletal muscles as well as carrying information from sensory organs such as the eye and ear. The autonomic nervous system serves the smooth muscles of the body (for example, around blood vessels), the cardiac muscle and glands. This autonomic nervous system is further divided into sympathetic and parasympathetic branches. The sympathetic branch is generally involved in the arousal of the organism and the expenditure of energy. For example, when confronted with a threat, the sympathetic branch will activate the so-called fight or flight response, resulting in an increase in heart rate and blood pressure, dilation of the pupils and an increase in the stress hormone cortisol. After the threat is handled, the parasympathetic branch will serve to relax the organism and conserve and store energy. Heart rate and blood pressure will decrease, pupils will constrict and cortisol levels will return to normal throughout the body.

The organization of the nervous system discussed above is the same basic arrangement found in other animals, although the human brain is different from that of other animals in its size and level of complexity. While the brains of other animals such as whales and elephants are larger, when corrected for body size the human brain is larger that that of any other animal. In addition, the level of complexity of the connections within the human brain is greater than in other animals. This combination of size and complexity enables the emergence of certain functions that, if not unique to humans, certainly characterize human mental life. As mentioned above, the theory of mind is an ability that seems to be associated with development of the frontal lobes. We must remember, however, that there is often no clear-cut dividing line between those species that possess a particular mental ability and those that do not. Nonhuman animals, such as chimpanzees, have demonstrated behaviors indicative of a theory of mind. These mental functions seem to exist on a continuum, and this gradation in ability is linked to the variation in level of complexity that exists between one species and another. Human brains share structural and physiological characteristics with the brains of lower animals, and these similarities are seen in the degree of overlap between human and nonhuman animals in behavioral and mental function.

Tools of Neuroscience

How do neuroscientists study the brain? How do they know which areas of the brain are involved in movement, vision, taste, memory or emotion? In the seventeenth century, early brain scientists like Thomas Willis tried to correlate observed behavior with damage to some part of the brain. Using autopsies and crude experiments on animals such as dogs, Willis and his colleagues made important observations regarding the involvement of the brain in mental and behavioral phenomena. Today, while more sophisticated methods are certainly used, the overall approach is similar in that an attempt is made to link some behavior (broadly defined) to a particular area of the brain that has been damaged, stimulated or whose activity is monitored by the experimenter. Many tools are at the modern-day neuroscientist's disposal. The following are just a few of these techniques that have enabled great progress to be made over the past three decades in our understanding of brain–behavior relationships.

Like Willis 350 years ago, today's brain scientist can use an autopsy to speculate on how a known mental or behavioral dysfunction present in a person might be related to brain damage observed during a post mortem examination. More typically, however, the modern neuroscientist will not wait for an autopsy to investigate the relationship between brain and behavior. Using animal subjects, various kinds of brain ablation techniques give clues to which brain areas are implicated in particular mental or behavioral events. Lesion studies involve damaging a particular brain structure (using relatively high levels of electrical current or chemicals) and inferring the role that structure has on behavior by observing how performance changes pre to post lesion. For example, a drug called kainic acid stimulates receptor sites for the neurotransmitter glutamate, causing those receptor sites to allow excessive amounts of calcium to enter the cell, resulting in cell death. When kainic acid is injected into the hippocampus, cells in this structure are damaged or die, and the researcher can begin to determine what role those cells play in learning, memory, or even a severe neurological disorder such as schizophrenia (Port and Seybold, 1995; Port, Sample and Seybold, 1991). Another method has the neuroscientist stimulate, using a mild electrical current, a particular brain structure and noting whether and in what ways behavior changes as a result of that stimulation.

The above kinds of procedures are typically performed on animals, most often on rats or mice, but sometimes on rabbits, cats or higher mammals. For human studies, these invasive procedures are not often used, although some of the same techniques, for example brain stimulation, can be used in a clinical setting in an attempt to treat certain neurological disorders such as Parkinson's disease. More typically, however, human studies involve various brain imaging procedures, whereby the neuroscientist can get a picture of what the brain looks like while the subject of the experiment is engaged in some kind of mental or behavioral task. Examples of these imaging tools include CT, MRI, PET, fMRI and SPECT.

Computerized tomography (CT) scans involve putting a person's head in a kind of tube which passes an X-ray beam through the head. A detector measures the amount of radioactivity that gets through the head and creates an X-ray like picture from the resulting measurements. These early brain scans provide relatively crude pictures of the brain, and can be used to locate lesions caused by strokes or brain tumors. A more detailed picture of the brain is provided by magnetic resonance imaging (MRI). These devices pass a strong magnetic field through the person's head, which causes nuclei in some atoms in the brain (particularly hydrogen atoms) to spin in a particular direction. A radio wave is then passed through the body, which causes these nuclei to give off specific radio waves which are detected by the MRI device and translated into a rather clear and precise picture of the brain (Carlson, 2007, p. 149).

More recently, new and improved brain scans which show the brain in action have been developed. These functional brain imaging techniques are useful in that researchers are able to picture the activity of different areas of the brain while the subject is performing some behavioral or mental task. One of the first functional scanning procedures was positron emission tomography (PET), in which the subject receives an injection of a radioactive substance such as glucose. The more active brain areas will absorb more of the glucose than the less active regions, and these differing absorption rates are translated into different colors by a computer. So the more active brain regions might be colored bright red or orange, while the less active areas are colored blue or brown. In this way, a neuroscientist might determine which brain areas are active (and therefore absorbing more glucose) while a person performs a mathematical calculation, or opens and closes their left hand, or makes a decision that involves a moral judgment. An even better functional scanning process is the functional magnetic resonance imaging procedure (fMRI). This is one of the newest scanning tools that measures different oxygen metabolism rates in various areas of the brain. Once again, any area that has a higher rate of metabolism is using more oxygen and is known to be active *vis-à-vis* an area with a low metabolism rate. These differing rates of oxygen metabolism are also translated via a computer into pictures with colors highlighting the areas of increased activity. The advantage of fMRI scans over the older PET scans is their higher degree of resolution and the speed at which the pictures of the brain are created (Carlson, 2007, p. 155).

The last scanning procedure to mention is single photon emission computed tomography (SPECT), a process similar to PET except that the radioactive tracer remains in the brain for several hours (unlike the short-acting tracer used in PET). This difference means that the tracer can be injected during a particular mental task, but the picture of brain activity during that task need not be taken until after the mental event is concluded. SPECT is used in the study of the brain's involvement in religious activity, and will be discussed in greater detail in Chapter 6.

How Does Neuroscience View Human Nature?

Many other tools exist in the neuroscientist's toolbox, including the recording of activity from a single neuron, tracing neural pathways using various stains, and examining the brain using high-power electron microscopes. Using these methods, neuroscientists have made great advances in our understanding of the brain and how it is involved in all of our behavior and mental life. In part because of these advances, the neuroscientist has developed a picture of human nature that is naturalistic, reductionistic, deterministic and monistic. The view sees humanity as part of nature itself. Human behavior and mental processes are understood as being determined by physical and chemical events in the brain. The mind, for many neuroscientists, is eliminated; the brain is all that remains. Once the brain is reduced to its basic components (neurons, neurotransmitters, ion channels and so on) and those elements studied in their entirety, these scientists believe we will know all there is to know about why we act, think, feel and believe the way we do. Others, while equally enthusiastic about the power of neuroscientific methods, are nevertheless more cautious in their speculations about whether we can ever know all there is to know about who we are as human beings by studying the nervous system. For these neuroscientists, reality, including the reality of human behavior and mind, is multileveled, and while neuroscience might make great advances in uncovering the mechanisms of the lower, more basic levels of human functioning, a complete view of the higher, more complex levels will remain beyond the gaze of neuroscience. For these scientists, science itself is limited in what it can tell us. In the opinion of these individuals, we are more than just a bunch of neurons, as the late Francis Crick once asserted. It is in this spirit of nonreductionism that this book examines what neuroscience, psychology and religion have to say about who we are as humans and why we behave the way we do.

Chapter 2

Psychology

Jennifer is a psychologist who works as a counselor in a community mental health clinic. She has a full load of clients, often treating as many as ten people during her long day. Each of her clients has a different kind of problem that is brought to the clinic. Some feel depressed, others are anxious about life in general. Many complain of having problems with a boss, spouse, friend or co-worker. Mary listens to her clients as they talk, administers various kinds of tests to try to assess the underlying problem, and sometimes gives advice. She also fills out a lot of paperwork. As much as half of her time is spent on paperwork that is related to the treatment of her clients, and to completing insurance forms so she can get paid for that service.

Kris is a psychologist who works for a large research university. She teaches two courses each semester for the psychology department, but most of her time is spent in a laboratory conducting research on the physiology of the visual system. Kris and the three graduate students who work for her in the lab are particularly interested in how the brain processes color. When she is not in the classroom or in the lab, Kris is writing papers about her research and submitting them to various scientific journals. It is particularly important for Kris to get her work published because she in applying for tenure at her university in two years, and she must have several of her papers in print for her to get tenure and keep her job. In addition, Kris must find sources of funding for her research. Her university has made it perfectly clear that she must obtain grants from private institutions or from the government, or she will not be tenured and will lose her job.

Mike is a psychologist who works for an electronics firm in its human resources department. Most of Mike's day consists of interviewing potential employees of the company, administering psychological tests to see which applicants would be good workers, and assessing existing workers to see how effective they are in their current positions. He has also, at times, been involved in negotiations between the electronics firm (which he represents) and the union that represents the hourly workers. While this aspect of his job is the most stressful and results in very long days of negotiating between the parties, it is the part of his work that he enjoys the most, and he often thinks about becoming a full-time negotiator after a few more years in the human resources department.

Each of these people does very different work; however, each went to graduate school in psychology and does work in the discipline of psychology. Psychology is a broad field that includes those who talk with and counsel others with problems (for example, clinical or counseling psychologists); those who work with children to understand their development (developmental psychologists); those who work in schools interacting with students and teachers to improve the learning environment (school or educational psychologists); those who work in industries of various kinds to help select employees, design machine-worker environments, and negotiate labor agreements (industrial/organizational psychologists); and those who teach in universities and do research in psychological science (experimental psychologists with various research interests).

While most people think of psychology as a part of the helping professions, a quick look at an introduction to psychology textbook (for example, Myers, 2005) will show just how diverse the discipline of psychology actually is, with chapters on biological psychology, research and statistics, developmental psychology, sensation and perception, consciousness, learning and memory, thinking and intelligence, motivation and emotion, personality, psychopathology, psychological therapy, and social psychology. It has been said that we live in a psychological society (Leahey, 2000, p. 544). The psychologist (particularly of the clinical or counseling variety) has replaced the rabbi, priest or clergyman as the person to go to with our concerns as well as for moral guidance. Psychologists are consulted on how to raise children, how to have a happy marriage, how to run a business effectively, how to control behavior in the classroom, and how we should think about and see ourselves. How did such a broad field like psychology develop? What were the intellectual sources of the discipline? How does psychology view human nature? How has psychology become such an influential force in our society? These are some of the questions addressed in this chapter.

The Beginnings of Psychology

The contemporary discipline of psychology is generally considered to have derived from two main sources: philosophy and science. In the case of the philosophical roots of modern psychology, we need to look to the Greek philosophers most notably Plato and Aristotle. With these two philosophers we see the beginnings of two distinct approaches to what knowledge is and how we obtain knowledge or learn. These two approaches, rationalism (Plato) and empiricism (Aristotle), helped shape not only subsequent philosophies, but also the discipline of psychology itself after it was founded in the late nineteenth century. Rationalism emphasized the importance of reason in the acquisition of knowledge, whereas empiricism emphasized the role of sensory data and experience. Another pair of tensions that emerged from the Greek philosophers is that of being versus becoming. Plato believed in the philosophy of being, which suggested that there are absolute, unchanging truths that can be known. Becoming is the philosophy that things in this world are always changing. 'The only constant in the universe is change' is a phrase to which the philosophers of becoming would agree.

These philosophical positions of rationalism and empiricism were also seen in the early Christian era and into the Middle Ages. Neoplatonism was advocated by the Christian philosopher/theologians Augustine (354–430) and Bonaventure (1221–1274), whereas Aristotelianism was the preferred philosophy of Aquinas (1225–1274). While not yet fully developed philosophies in the Middle Ages, rationalism and empiricism can nevertheless be used as a basic way to distinguish the approaches of the medieval philosophers as they considered the problems of knowledge, learning, memory, behavior and so on.

Renaissance and Enlightenment Influences on Psychology and the Rise of Naturalism

In the sixteenth through eighteenth centuries, these approaches emphasizing reason and experience became fully developed philosophies of rationalism and empiricism. As a formal philosophical approach, rationalism argued that all knowledge is the result of a rational analysis of sensory evidence. The mind is structured so that sensory data are organized in a manner that can be interpreted and understood, and these mental structures exist *a priori* to sensory experience. Empiricism, on the other hand, argued that evidence of the senses is the primary source of all knowledge and that all intellectual processes must use sensory evidence to form truthful propositions about the real world. Neither rationalism nor empiricism at this time rejected mental processes as being important in the acquisition of knowledge, nor did either approach believe that sensory data were unimportant. They did differ, however, in the emphasis they placed on sensory experience or reason and cognitive processes, with empiricism emphasizing experience over reason, and rationalism reason over experience. Major empiricist philosophers during this time included John Locke (1632–1704), who believed that the mind is a *tabula rasa*, or blank slate, written upon by experience, George Berkeley (1685–1753), who famously suggested that objects do not have an existence apart from our perception of them, and David Hume (1711–1776), who emphasized the primacy of sensory data over ideas. Important rationalist philosophers from this era included René Descartes (1596–1650), who made a clear distinction between the material body and the immaterial (and much more important) mind or soul, Gottfried von Leibniz (1646–1716), who suggested that the mind contains innate potentials and tendencies much like a veined block of marble has internal lines of cleavage which predispose it to be sculpted into some shapes more easily than others, and Immanuel Kant (1724–1808), who argued that certain logical functions (for example, causation) are imposed upon evidence of the senses, not derived from evidence of the senses as some of the empiricist philosophers suggested.

While the philosophies of rationalism and empiricism were becoming formalized during the sixteenth through eighteenth centuries, another significant development was the growing emphasis upon naturalism, and it was this viewpoint that effected the greatest change in how humans saw their world and themselves. Naturalism describes nature as operating like a machine. In fact, the metaphor of the machine became increasingly used, beginning in the seventeenth century with the writings of Thomas Hobbes (1588–1679), Claude Helvétius (1715–1771) and Julien de la Mettrie (1709–1751). While Descartes made a clear separation between the material (and mechanical) body and the immaterial soul or mind, Helvétius collapsed the distinction by arguing that matter itself is endowed with the power of thought, so there is no need for a spiritual or immaterial soul. One only needs a brain to think, reason, make judgments, and so on. The characteristic faculties of the soul or mind are actually, according to Helvétius, powers of the material brain. This conclusion was based, in part, on experimental work done about a hundred years earlier by Thomas Willis (1621–1675). Dissecting the brains of deceased individuals who had well-known behavioral, cognitive and personality abnormalities while living suggested to Willis that the qualities of humanness generally ascribed to the soul were actually abilities derived from the brain itself (Zimmer, 2004).

Helvétius's view had earlier been applied to society as a whole by Hobbes, who declared that man was a social machine and that the laws of society operate like the laws of physics. This machine metaphor was vigorously advocated by La Mettrie, who wrote in *L'Homme Machine* (1748) that man's soul was an enlightened machine. Both body and soul are machines, and the proper functioning of the soul, according to La Mettrie, depends on the correct operation of the brain, as well as of the whole body.

With this rise of mechanism and naturalism, especially in the human sciences, came a secularization of knowledge. People were less likely to be seen as souls in need of salvation, and more likely understood as machines to be studied and explained. But if humans are mere machines, what is the ground for moral values and meaning? If, as the Marquis de Sade suggested, we should pursue pleasure, and if it is nature's way for the strong to rule the weak, upon what is any system of morality based? This is the fundamental problem for a naturalistic *philosophy* (as opposed to a naturalistic *methodology*) that believes humans are on earth by chance and that there is no purpose for our existence; we merely live (ideally, in the pursuit of pleasure and in the domination of the weak), and then die. It was this naturalistic or materialistic view of humanity (the machine metaphor) that developed in the sixteenth through eighteenth centuries and influenced both the natural sciences and the human sciences like psychology that were founded in the nineteenth century.

Psychology's Roots in Science

While one branch of psychology's family tree can be traced through philosophy, the other major contributor to the founding of psychology was science, particularly the sciences of physiology and physics in the nineteenth century. One of the specific developments in physiology that was instrumental in the founding of psychology was the work of Hermann Helmholtz (1821–1894), who, among other significant discoveries, was able to measure the speed of an electrical impulse as it is conducted down the axon of a brain cell (neuron). The importance of this work was that the speed was found to be relatively slow, less that 50 m per second, well below the previously estimated velocity approaching the speed of sound, if not of light. Because the speed was slow enough to be measurable using nineteenth-century equipment, this opened up the possibility of measuring mental and behavioral acts, which were included in the subject matter of the earliest psychologists.

Another significant scientific development that influenced the founding of psychology as a discipline was the attempt to determine how many, if any, of the mind's faculties are localizable to specific brain regions. In the late eighteenth and early nineteenth centuries, Franz Joseph Gall (1758–1828) and Johann Spurzheim

(1776–1832) promoted the 'science of mind' known as phrenology. Phrenology was predicated on three fundamental principles. First, the exterior surface of the skull corresponds to the interior surface of the brain. Second, the mind is analyzable into separate and independent mental faculties, such as benevolence, cautiousness, hope, acquisitiveness, secretiveness, language, time, causality and order. Third, these faculties are localizable onto specific regions or areas of the brain, and excess in brain structure corresponds to excess in the mental faculty. (Deficits in the brain at a specific location also correspond to impairments in that localized mental faculty.) It was thought by the phrenologists that one could 'read' another person's cognitive ability and/or personality traits by feeling that person's head for the bumps and depressions in the skull that correspond to the underlying excesses or deficiencies in brain.

Phrenology became an incredibly popular form of 'psychological' testing. Couples had phrenological readings in order to determine whether they were suitable for marriage. Potential employees were required by future employers to have a phrenologist do a reading to see whether they were an appropriate fit for a job. Phrenology was a craze in Europe as well as in the United States, and the last journal of phrenology did not cease publication until the early part of the twentieth century.

While the foundations of phrenology were unsound (for example, the overlying skull does not reflect the underlying surface of the brain), the movement began an attempt by brain scientists to see to what extent mental faculties or functions are in fact localizable to specific brain regions. The spirit of the times, or *Zeitgeist*, was moving the mind away from a Cartesian concept of an immaterial soul toward a material view of the mind, and phrenology was both a cause and a symptom of this *Zeitgeist*.

Brain scientists came down on both sides of the question. Pierre Flourens (1794–1867) concluded that the mind is a unity, and that only a few gross functions (for example, movement) were localizable to rather large brain regions (for example, the cerebellum). Others, however, such as Paul Broca (1824–1880), provided evidence that there was greater specificity of function to a given brain area than Flourens suspected. Broca was able to identify an area in the brain that seemed to be responsible for the very human characteristic of speech. This debate about the localization of brain function carried over into the twentieth century with the work of Karl Lashley (1890–1958), who argued, based on his experiments in animals, that the mental function of memory is spread throughout the cortex, but that certain aspects of the memory (for example, the visual component) is localized in a rather circumscribed area of the brain.

Other developments in the study of light and sound, sensation, reflex action, and movement also occupied the research time of physicists and physiologists. It was the work of physicist turned philosopher turned physiologist Gustav Fechner (1801–1887) that brought the methods of nineteenth-century science to the study of the issue that had been a problem for philosophers since the time of the Greeks. The philosophical issue Fechner addressed was the relationship between the mind (or soul) and the body.

Fechner was a professor of physics at the University of Leipzig when he began to question the rising tide of materialism and naturalism he saw not only in physics, but in other disciplines as well. Perhaps as a partial result of this tension, he became ill and almost an invalid in 1839, resigning his professorship and cutting himself off from most people. He did recover in 1846, and began to give lectures on topics that interested him, topics such as the philosophy of nature, life and death, and the body–soul relationship. Fechner contrasted his post-illness worldview, which he called the 'Day View', with the purely materialistic and reductionistic perspective he saw developing in the natural sciences. This materialistic worldview, which he termed the 'Night View', limited human knowledge to a material reality and was pessimistic, cold and impersonal. Fechner's Day View was his attempt to explain both material and mental reality and to unite the real world of people with science, not eliminate that subjective reality, as materialism tended to do (Heidelberger, 2004). Psychophysics was Fechner's attempt to verify empirically the relationship between the physical world and our subjective response to that physical world – in other words, the relationship between bodily stimulation and mental response to that stimulation. The body and the mind to Fechner are one thing viewed from two different perspectives, much like a coin can be viewed from either of two sides. Also like a coin, however, only one side is observable at a time. One can take the perspective of the physical body or the perspective of the mind, but not both simultaneously (Heidelberger, 2004).

The New Psychology

Fechner's psychophysics became a primary subject matter for the early psychologists as they tried to develop ways to measure mental activity and responses. It was Wilhelm Wundt (1832–1920), however, who intentionally set out to found a new discipline devoted to studying the content of mental activity or consciousness using the tools of nineteenth-century physiology. This new physiological psychology, founded in 1879 in Leipzig, Germany, quickly attracted students from around Europe and the United States. While American students went to Leipzig to study under Wundt, they returned to the United States with alternative ideas of what this new discipline of psychology would study and what the methods of this psychology would be. The psychology that emerged in the United States was heavily influenced by Darwin's evolutionary theory, and began to investigate not the content, but the function of mind and consciousness. What purpose does consciousness serve? What adaptive advantage does it provide those organisms in which it evolved?

A leader of this functionalistic psychology in the United States was William James (1842–1910), who became the most influential academic American psychologist for several decades, and whose work is cited even today in the current literature. His most significant publications were *The Principles of Psychology*, published in 1890, and *The Varieties of Religious Experience*, which consisted of lectures on psychology and religion given by James and published in 1902. James's psychology was pragmatic, functional, and covered a wide range of topics including emotion, attention, memory, habit and religion (both healthy and unhealthy).

While the functional psychology of James and others (for example, James Angell and John Dewey) was influenced by Darwin's evolutionary theory, its primary subject matter was still consciousness. Psychology from its founding had always patterned itself after the natural sciences of physics and physiology, but having a subject matter like consciousness, a phenomenon an increasing number of psychologists believed to be closed to scientific investigation, required a change in direction. The change was not, however, toward new methods in which to study consciousness. The change was toward a new subject matter, one that could be studied using the tools of the natural sciences, and that new subject matter for psychology was behavior.

Psychological Science in the Twentieth Century

With the publication of 'Psychology as the behaviorist views it' in 1913, John Watson (1878–1958) heralded the beginning of a completely new kind of psychology, one that would be objective, scientific, and much more closely tied to the evolutionary theory of Charles Darwin. In the article, which appeared in the journal *Psychological Review*, Watson declared that psychology's subject matter, mental phenomena, was incompatible with scientific method because of its lack of objectivity, and it was for that reason that there had not been much progress within psychology since its founding in 1879. Because behavior is public and objective, it does lend itself to the methods of the natural sciences, and if those methods are used, a dramatic increase in psychological understanding would, according to Watson, result. Among the important elements of behaviorism as a movement within psychology was evolutionary theory. One of the basic tenets of behaviorism was that animal and human behavior could be studied using the same methods. Darwin's theory suggested a basic continuity of physiology and behavior among the species, so studying the behavior of rats or pigeons was justified on the principle that insights gained from research on those species could be generalized to human behavior. An additional contributing influence on early behaviorism was the work of experimentalists in Russia such as Ivan Sechenov and Ivan Pavlov, both of whom emphasized the importance of environmental stimuli on the elicitation and production of behavior. This deterministic and mechanistic view of the causes of behavior was widely accepted by behaviorists in the twentieth century.

While behaviorism is often associated with the work of B.F. Skinner (1904–1990), there were actually different kinds of behaviorism ranging from Skinner's experimental analysis of behavior, which looked for the functional relationships between apparent environmental stimuli and observable behavior, to Edward Tolman's (1886–1959) cognitive behaviorism, which referred to variables that intervene between the observable stimulus and response. The use of these intervening variables, such as expectancies and cognitive maps, made Tolman's 'purposive behaviorism' a harbinger of cognitive psychology which emerged on the scene in the 1960s and 1970s. Despite their differences, behaviorists from Skinner to Tolman shared a dedication to methodological naturalism, the belief that the causes of behavior are to be found in natural mechanisms, and that the scientific method is the best approach to uncover those mechanisms. Behaviorists also shared a basic understanding of human nature, one which viewed the human person as, to one degree or another, a machine whose behavior can be understood in a deterministic, reductionistic and materialistic fashion. While traditional Western views of humanity and human behavior might emphasize freedom and responsibility, the typical behavioral view (especially in Skinner's hands) emphasized control via the environment, manipulation, and a lack of behavioral freedom or responsibility.

The behavioral approach in psychology – which emphasized the study of behavior, and the neglect, at least for many behaviorists, of any interest in consciousness or mind – was challenged in the 1960s and 1970s with the emergence of cognitive psychology and its emphasis on the study of mental phenomena such as thinking, reasoning, memory and decision making. Heavily influenced by information theory and the work of Norbert Wiener, Claude Shannon and Warren Weaver, cognitive psychology introduced the concept of information processing into experimental psychology. People became channels of information, and the importance of how stimuli are encoded by the receiving person was emphasized. Cognitive psychology was also influenced by the growing field of computer science, and the computer quickly became a model of how information is processed by humans.

The traditional view of this portion of psychology's history suggests that a cognitive revolution took place where the old and no longer adequate behavioral paradigm was replaced by the newer and better cognitivism. This way of understanding the transition from one approach in psychology to another has been challenged by Thomas Leahey, who questions, first, the assumption that behaviorism represented a true paradigm in psychology, second, the belief that cognitivism itself is a new paradigm, and third, that a revolution actually occurred in psychology (Leahey, 1992). Leahey argues that both behaviorism and cognitivism are continuations of the trend toward naturalism, mechanism and reductionism characteristic of psychology (and science in general) since its founding. While cognitive psychology might recognize the importance of consciousness and mind, aspects of human experience and reality often ignored by the behaviorists, it nevertheless is mechanistic, naturalistic and generally deterministic in its approach to mental activity and consciousness. The mind is, after all, like a computer to the cognitivists, and a computer is certainly a machine whose functioning is very much determined by how it is programmed. Human information processing is also machine-like and highly determined by the kind of program provided by our biology embedded within a particular environment. The picture of human nature, then, that emerges in psychological science is essentially one of naturalistic forces (biology, physiology, chemistry, environment and so on) influencing behavior and mental activity in a fundamentally deterministic and mechanistic way.

The Psychological Society

After the First World War and then again after the Second World War, psychology experienced rapid growth in its influence on American society. The use of psychological testing, including intelligence tests, to place recruits effectively during the wars was extended to the extensive testing of children as well as adults after the wars to determine their intellectual and/or mental capabilities. Clinical psychology became dominant within the discipline of psychology after the Second World War with the development of the scientist-practitioner model of training psychologists to provide mental health care. In addition, industrial/organizational psychology, the use of psychological principles within a business or industrial setting, matured as American businesses experienced tremendous growth during the postwar years. In short, American psychology became much more applied beginning during the middle portion of the twentieth century. This increasing influence of applied psychology (over the more traditional and original experimental psychology of Wundt and James) resulted in disagreements between those who promoted a psychology that would be 'useful' and those who wanted psychology to remain a more 'academic' subject. While those who longed to keep psychology within the more pure sciences succeeded in founding their own organizations (for example, the American Psychological Society, now called the Association for Psychological Science, founded in 1988 by psychologists who were disenchanted by the trend toward the professionalization of psychology emphasized within the older and larger American Psychological Association), psychology as a discipline nevertheless became more and more applied during the last half of the twentieth century. At least within the minds of the general population, psychology is thought of as one of the helping professions. Jennifer in the introduction to this chapter is the quintessential psychologist. She sits in an office and listens to 'clients' as they talk about their problems. She may, depending upon her theoretical orientation, offer advice, assign homework or just listen, but she is nevertheless helping another person with a problem (for example, marriage, work-related or parental).

Psychology today, in the words of psychologist Paul Vitz, has become a kind of religion in which the self is worshiped (Vitz, 1977, p. 9). The psychologist, especially the clinician, has replaced the priest, rabbi or clergyman as the person to whom people turn in times of trouble. It is the psychologist who provides advice on the raising of children, who assesses the compatibility of a couple for marriage, who offers suggestions to teachers on how to handle a difficult student in the classroom, who assists in selecting the correct person for a job at a company and then tests to see how that person is performing on the job. It is the psychologist, and other therapists, who rush to scenes of trauma (real or imagined) expecting to assist the victims of that trauma (again real or imagined) through their grief. If no signs of grief are present, too often that lack of emotion is seen as an indication that the grief is being 'repressed', only to be released, if not treated, at a later time and in an unhealthy way. It is the expert on the self who is the high priest in a society that worships the individual self. (Nothing can be worse in such a society than 'low self-esteem', which is blamed for low grades in school, drug abuse, teenage pregnancy, increased violence and every other societal problem. In some classrooms in the United States, mistakes on a test or paper are no longer marked with a red pen because red is 'judgmental' and 'stressful'. Instead, more 'pleasant-feeling' colors like pink and purple are used because they are seen as being more 'compassionate'; Will, 2005.)

Perhaps it was inevitable that psychology would become such an important part of our society. Over the course of the last 400 years or so, there has been a steady movement away from a religious and metaphysical outlook on life and toward a more mechanistic understanding of nature and humanity. This trend toward mechanization and naturalism has resulted in great success in the sciences, the approach to knowledge that seeks naturalistic explanations. However, 'As religious and metaphysical traditions have been eroded by mechanistic science, people have turned to science for moral guidance, and this has led them, inevitably, to psychology, the science of individual action' (Leahey, 2000, p. 545). Instead of an inner quest for God, Americans at least undertake a quest for the self, and it is the psychologist who is seen as the guru on that quest. It is the psychologist (in the home, in the office, in the classroom) who can lead the seeker to inner truth and high self-esteem, the only truth possible, and the only valid goal within a culture that places such an emphasis on the individual.

Levels of Nature and Levels of Psychology

From its beginning, psychology has wanted to be like the natural sciences of physics and physiology. (It is sometimes said that psychology suffers from 'physics envy'.) This desire to be like the natural sciences and to study behavior and mental processing (a standard definition of psychology found in any introductory psychology textbook) as a natural science raises important questions. One of those questions is to what extent the human sciences like psychology can be studied successfully in the same way as nature (Bhaskar, 1998, p. 1). Are the subject matters of psychology and physics (or biology or chemistry) so different that different methods are required? Another way on putting this is to ask whether methodology (the way to study something) is dependent of ontology (the essential nature of that something).

Philosopher Roy Bhaskar and others talk about the stratification of reality, by which they mean there are ordered and hierarchical layers or strata to a particular phenomenon in reality. One might arrive at an explanation for one layer, but there are other, more basic and deeper layers that can always be studied and explained. For example, consider the phenomenon of an illness such as schizophrenia (McGrath, 2002, p. 229). Illnesses can be understood at the rather basic level of *pathology*. What is the abnormality in function and/or structure of an organ or system? In schizophrenia there is evidence that the brain is affected as indicated by an increase in ventricular volume and abnormalities in connections within the prefrontal cortex and between this frontal lobe structure and other areas of the brain. An illness can also be understood and described at the higher level of *impairment*. There are certain symptoms of schizophrenia, such as hallucinations, delusions, disordered thinking, social withdrawal and flattening of affect, that impact not just a single organ or system, but the entire organism. Third, an illness can be understood at the level of *activity*, whereby the symptoms mentioned above have a detrimental effect on the person's behavior and interaction with others and the environment. Clearly, a person with schizophrenia who hears voices that are not really there and thinks the CIA is trying to kill them is going to have a very difficult time interacting with others and with the environment. Finally, an illness such as schizophrenia can be understood by its effect at the *participation* level of analysis. The illness impacts the victim's ability to hold down a job, care for one's family, take part in worship services, and so on.

Each of these hierarchical levels may require a specific method of study appropriate to the nature of the phenomena at that stratum. Methods appropriate for study at the pathology level are not necessarily correct for investigation of the illness at the participation level. While the deficits seen at the participation level are affected by the deficits in the lower levels (for example, activity), they cannot be reduced to 'nothing but' those lower-level deficiencies. In this regard, the hallucinations and delusions seen in schizophrenia at the level of impairment are said to emerge from the abnormalities in the more basic level of brain pathology; however, these symptoms and signs of schizophrenia cannot be said, according to this stratification of reality approach, to be reduced to those lower-strata pathologies.

What are the implications of this stratification of reality for psychology? Because reality is multileveled, it is understandable that there should be multiple kinds of sciences with multiple methodologies to study that reality. The methods and approach represented in the psychological sciences are appropriate for investigations at the psychological level of reality. In a similar manner, the methods and approach of the biological sciences are proper for investigation at the biological level, and the physical sciences use methods suitable to the physical level of reality. In studying an illness like schizophrenia, biology will be used to study the basic level of underlying neural pathology, psychology will be used to investigate at the level of activity, and perhaps the methods of the social sciences will be used to investigate schizophrenia at the higher level of participation. The stratification of reality demands that various approaches be employed and consulted for a complete (or as complete as we can reasonably expect) understanding of any illness.

Some in the natural sciences, and even in the psychological sciences, have suggested that psychology can be reduced to biology, in that all behavior and mental processing is based upon biological (that is, nervous system) activity. In turn, biology can be reduced to chemistry, and chemistry is ultimately reducible to physics. If this is true, only one level of analysis and one methodology is appropriate. Bhaskar and others, however, suggest that this reductionistic view of human behavior, mental life, consciousness and human nature itself is wrong. Yes, there are more basic levels below psychology in the hierarchy or stratification of reality and the sciences. But the stratification or levels view of reality rejects the notion that all of the levels are reducible to the basic level. When an explanation for a particular phenomenon is found at one level or stratum, another deeper and more basic explanation can be sought that complements and reinforces, not replaces, the higher-level account (Collier, 1994, p. 110).

Within psychology, there are levels of explanation as well. Physiological psychology, which is the study of the biological bases of behavior, might be the most basic level within psychological science. Other levels above physiological psychology might include cognitive psychology, developmental psychology and social psychology, to name just a few. Study of social behavior, developmental patterns, cognition, as well as the function of the nervous system, is necessary for a well-rounded understanding of human behavior and mental life. Some voices in psychology are suggesting that the way psychology studies a particular aspect of mental processing or behavior (for example, decision making) must change to include more interaction, not only among the various subfields of psychology, but also across several disciplines. There is a social and emotional component to decision making (for example, social intuitionist model), a developmental component to decision making (for example, the development of a Theory of Mind), as well as clear brain (for example, amygdala and prefrontal cortex) involvement in decision making. Each of these specialty areas in psychological science, and others, needs to be considered when studying that particular mental ability. The same could be said of intelligence, reasoning, memory and many other behavioral and mental abilities and functions.

So psychological science is an appropriate approach to studying natural phenomena from the psychological level of reality. While explanations from this level can be reinforced by explanations from a lower level (for example, biology), the higher-level explanations remain in force as adjuncts or complements. Reality is complex. Human behavior and mental activity are part of that complex reality, and it takes many different approaches from a variety of disciplines to get a full (or as near as we can get at the present time) understanding of these multifaceted phenomena. As such, psychological science, incomplete though it is, has a vital role to play, along with biology, chemistry, the neurosciences and other natural and human sciences, in understanding who we are as human beings, and how and why we behave and think the way we do.

Chapter 3

Religion

The Sistine chapel in the Vatican houses some of the greatest art in the Western world. Examples of these classic pieces of art are the frescos on the ceiling of the chapel. There, Michelangelo painted scenes from Genesis beginning with the 'Separation of Light and Darkness' and moving to the 'Drunkenness of Noah'. Included among these scenes is the 'Creation of Adam', in which the divine finger is reaching out to touch the finger of Adam and to bestow upon the first man a spirit or soul. Adam is different from the rest of creation; he is made in the image of God, the *imago Dei*. A few years ago, the frescos of the Sistine chapel were restored and cleaned. After removing centuries of dirt and grime, bright colors emerged and new, clearer views of the paintings were possible. In the 'Creation of Adam', God is surrounded by the host of heaven, including Eve and what some art historians have identified as the Christ child. But the heavenly host and God himself are enclosed in a wispy kind of structure, a part of the painting that was not as apparent before the restoration. As this structure came into clearer view, some observers suggested that the formation resembled a brain. The cerebral hemispheres seem to surround God and the host of heaven. Could Michelangelo be suggesting something from this portrayal of God? Could he be suggesting perhaps that what God is giving to Adam as depicted in this picture is somehow related to the functioning of the brain? Could the spirit or soul bestowed upon Adam at this instant be dependent on the human brain for its existence?

As we will discuss in a later chapter, there is increasing evidence from the neurosciences and from psychology that indeed our soul (or self, personhood, consciousness and so on) is highly dependent on the brain and nervous system. Could Michelangelo have anticipated the findings of twenty-first-century science almost 500 years earlier? Perhaps we will never know what Michelangelo intended when he painted those great scenes in the early sixteenth century. What we do know, however, is that Michelangelo's masterpiece does depict a central event in the Judeo-Christian religious tradition. What does it mean to be created in the image of God, to have the *imago Dei*? What does having God's image mean for us as we relate to the rest of creation, most importantly perhaps, to our fellow human beings? What does being created with the *imago Dei* mean as far as our human nature is concerned? These are some of the questions raised by religion, and they are also related to the picture of human nature imagined by neuroscience and psychology.

After discussing some of the fundamentals of neuroscience and psychology in Chapters 1 and 2 (including their views of human nature), we need to do the same for religion. What is religion? Where did it come from, and why does it seem to be a universal characteristic of human societies? Is there a difference between religion and spirituality? How might we be able to measure these concepts? What is a religious view (particularly Christian) of nature and of human nature?

One is tempted to think that there is general agreement among scholars about what science is and about what constitutes religion. In fact, there is much discussion about what these terms mean. Many different disciplines might be considered examples of science. The most obvious, perhaps, are physics, chemistry and biology. Most people would agree that individuals working in these fields are doing science, and that the results of research in these areas represents true scientific knowledge. Other disciplines, however, are less obviously scientific in their approach. As we saw in Chapter 2, psychology desperately wants to be considered a science, and some of its sub-disciplines (for example, physiological psychology and cognitive psychology) would by most standards be considered science. Other sub-areas in psychology, however, might not reach the standard of true science in the opinion of biologists, chemists or physicists. The point is that there is no consensus definition of what science is or what disciplines are scientific.

It is also the case that there is much disagreement about the nature of religion. While most would agree that Christianity, Judaism, Hinduism and Islam are clearly examples of world religions, there is less agreement about New Age, Native, or even Buddhism. And within these broader categories, there are questions about the religious legitimacy of specific sects or behaviors within the religious groups (for example, serpent handling, speaking in tongues, visions). Just as there is no agreed-upon definition of science, there seems to be no agreement about the definition of religion. An anthropologist's characterization of religion will no doubt be different from the definition given by a psychologist or that of a theologian. Nevertheless, in order to think about the relations between neuroscience, psychology and religion, we need to consider the nature of religion just as we did in the first two chapters when we looked at the nature of neuroscience and psychology respectively. In addition, we must consider whether religion is different from or the same thing as spirituality. Recent self-report surveys of adolescents and young adults indicate that their spirituality is important to them even as their interest in traditional religions wanes. But just what is meant by spirituality, and how different is it from religiosity? In this chapter, we will look at these questions and others as we lay the necessary ground work in order to understand the importance and relevance of recent findings in neuroscience and psychology for religious faith.

What is a Religion?

Perhaps it is understandable, or even necessary, that any discussion of religion from a psychological perspective begin with how William James defined religion. James was a philosopher who was instrumental in developing academic psychology in the United States. Working at the end of the nineteenth century, James became an advocate for the development of a new discipline, an experimental psychology, which would attempt to find answers to the questions about human knowledge, behavior, thinking and emotion contemplated for centuries by individuals such as Plato, Aristotle and Descartes. These answers, however, would not be found via discussion and debate, but through the experimental approach developed beginning in the seventeenth century and by taking advantage of the new instrumentation and technologies physiologists and physicists created in the nineteenth century. In his classic work *The Varieties of Religious Experience* (which consisted of a series of lectures given on natural theology or how science and religion might be seen to 'fit' together), James defined religion as 'the feelings, acts, and experiences of individual men in their solitude, so far as they apprehend themselves to stand in relation to whatever they may consider the divine' (James, 1902/1999, p. 36). A number of difficulties with this definition immediately come to mind. Specifically, how are we to define the terms in James's definition, terms such as 'feelings', 'acts', 'experiences' and 'divine'?

The idea that one can even come up with a true definition of religion is a Western notion. Some argue that defining religion is impossible, and the best one can do is try to recognize various traditions, movements, behaviors and so on that people over time and across cultures have used. Others suggest, however, that all religions minimally involve beliefs and behaviors with a supernatural orientation (that is, directed to spiritual beings or to a supernatural realm) (McGrath, 1999, p. 30). Of course, even this attempt to define religion raises further questions regarding the definition of belief, or what is meant by 'supernatural'. We can even ask the question 'What is God?', because religions can entail theism, deism, polytheism, panentheism, pantheism, monotheism and so on. Faith is also an important part of religion for many individuals. But again, we can think about different kinds of faith – for example, faith in a person, faith in a particular idea, faith in some specific way of life (Drees, 1996, p. 29) – or different 'definitions' of faith (Midgley, 2002, p. 16).

Some have tried to define religion on the basis of certain intellectual content. For example, a religion in this view would have a set of positions regarding the nature of God, salvation, eschatology and so on. The positions, of course, would be potentially different from one religion to the next, but from this perspective, religion consists of a collection of important intellectual beliefs that relate to the transcendent and/or to spiritual beings. Another way of defining religion focuses not on beliefs, but on the function of religion. What do religious beliefs or practices do for the individual? What purpose do they serve? Efforts to understand religion using this kind of approach would emphasize the role that religion plays in bringing communities of people together, giving those communities a common purpose, and the potential value of community in communal or individual health. Still others might emphasize the role of institutions in a definition of religion.

While a consensus definition of religion might not be possible, perhaps religion is one of those phenomena in which 'We know it when we see it.' For example, we believe that we know Christianity when we see it being expressed. (Although even this simple statement is questionable in that some Christian sects and denominations do not consider members of other Christian groups or denominations 'authentic' or 'true' Christians.) Nevertheless, in this chapter we are going to limit our discussion to Christianity. The reason for this is that Christianity is the religion (however we care to define that term) of the author and of most of the intended audience of this book. It is also the form of religious expression in which the most effort has been expended trying to integrate it with science. It is not necessarily the case that other forms of religion cannot be brought into discussion with the findings of science; for example, some effort has been made to relate science with Islam (see Dhanani, 2002, pp. 73–92). It is simply the case that the great majority of science and religion discussions have considered the relationship between science and Christianity.

What is the Origin of Religion?

Religious belief is widespread within the human species. While the form of religious expression will necessarily be different from culture to culture, the fact that the worship of someone or some thing is found in virtually all peoples suggests that religious belief is a universal characteristic of human societies. What accounts for the fact that people across the globe tend to engage in rituals, perform behaviors, experience emotions and hold particular ideas that are considered religious in nature?

One answer to this question is provided by saying that the God of creation made himself known to his creation. This revelation came to select individuals such as Abraham, through whom, and in response to God, the Israelites developed the rituals, practices and legal obligations that form so much of the Judeo-Christian tradition. Or, in the case of Islam, Allah communicated through Mohammad, and as a result, the basic principles of that religion were instantiated. These religious beliefs, doctrines and practices are provided via supernatural revelations. They come from outside of human experience, and are therefore independent of human construction.

An alternative view of the origin of these religious beliefs and practices argues that they are not independent of human experience, but are in fact human inventions. This is the position taken by E.O. Wilson in his controversial but influential book *Concilience*, published in 1998. In his book, Wilson, a biologist from Harvard University, lays out his goal, which is to try to unify knowledge under a few general laws and principles. Specifically, Wilson believes that all human knowledge, including ethics, morality and religion, can ultimately be reduced to biology, chemistry and physics. Religious commandments, beliefs, practices and so on are not given from the outside (that is, from God, Allah, or any other transcendental source); they are merely human inventions that can be explained by appealing to certain biological principles such as natural selection.

In the 1970s, Wilson became famous (some would say infamous) for developing and promoting the movement known as sociobiology. Sociobiology tried to understand (and perhaps explain away) social behaviors such as helping others, mate selection and parenting by arguing that the behaviors reflect the influence of biology on the organism. Many, however, saw in Wilson's views a rigid biological determinism that de-emphasized the role of the environment and learning on behavior in favor of a strong (perhaps, some thought, exclusive) role of genetics. One of the reasons that Wilson's sociobiology was rejected, particularly by those coming from the political left, was that the emphasis on genetic determinism over environmental manipulation raised fears of a new form of eugenics. As a result, sociobiology dropped out of favor among many academics.

In the 1990s, a new version of sociobiology emerged which has, to this point, avoided many of the negative connotations associated with sociobiology. The new approach is called evolutionary psychology (see Chapter 8 of this book), and sees all human behavior as ultimately resulting from evolutionary forces (for example, random variation and natural selection). It is from the perspective of evolutionary psychology that Wilson wrote *Concilience*. Ethics and morality are seen by evolutionary psychologists as behaviors that have been selected via evolution because they serve to increase the survival advantage of those who perform the behaviors. Telling the truth, for example, has been evolutionarily selected because those individuals exhibiting truthful behaviors in the past were more likely to survive and reproduce than those individuals who told lies. Another version suggests that it is the genes for telling the truth, not the individuals themselves, that have been selected and have been passed onto the next generation. The reason why telling the truth might be a selective advantage (either via genes or individual selection) is because for individuals to survive, they must join together with other individuals for mutual protection and for hunting and gathering purposes. In other words, individuals must join together and form a larger group or society, and in order to form these societies, the individuals in them must be able to trust each other. Societies where the individual members do not trust each other will not be able to join forces to reap the advantages of the larger group. For example, if the individual group members do not trust the others in the group that the meat of the kill will be shared equally among all those who helped in the hunt, there is no incentive for them to work together, even though doing so will make for an easier kill of a larger prey and potentially more food for each. It is through these kinds of connections that societies get larger and stronger.

In order to form these organized bans, however, certain rules develop to help insure that trust will be maintained. Evolutionary psychology suggests, for example, that an individual who 'cheats' another will likely be shunned by the community. Such shunning helps to guarantee that future instances of such 'cheating' will not occur, upon penalty of being kicked out of the group and depending solely upon oneself. In this way, honesty is selected for and the genes that promote honest behavior are passed on to the next generation. Gradually, over many thousands of years, these selected behaviors become what we now know as ethical principles. It is good to be honest. It is ethical to tell the truth. These ideas, however, come not from outside human experience, but from the very biology of humanity itself.

In a similar way, religious ideas and beliefs are developed via evolutionary processes. For example, the religious belief in an afterlife might have developed as a result of the human mind's need for emotional comfort in the face of our own mortality. As the mind evolved in complexity to the point where recognition of eventual death was possible, the mind needed a way to make this mortality less unbearable. The result was the belief in life after death, an eternal existence after this earthly body dies (Boyer, 2001, p. 19).

One of the world's foremost evolutionary zoologists is Richard Dawkins of the University of Oxford. Dawkins famously likens belief in God and other religious tenets to a mind virus. Why do the vast majority of people believe there is a God? Not, according to Dawkins, because they have thought about the issue and come to a reasonable conclusion. As an atheist, Dawkins believes there is no God, so it is not possible to come to a reasonable conclusion that God exists. So, if one does believe in God, it must be because the God virus has survival value, as does the belief in an afterlife as discussed above. Like other viruses that infect the body or a computer, however, this mind virus is harmful, unhealthy, and should be eliminated. One of the roles of science is to help get rid of these mind viruses. Science is an example of a positive or useful program that spreads from one mind to another on the basis of good methodological standards such as testability and evidential support (Dawkins, 2003, p. 138). Dawkins seems blissfully unaware that religious beliefs (or theories) are also subjected to methodological standards such as evidential support. He also does not recognize that his own atheism can be considered a mind virus. What is a 'good' mind program and what is a 'harmful' mind virus is not really something that can be determined empirically, despite Dawkins's reliance on scientific methodology. Essentially, Dawkins relies on the old standby argument based on subjectivity: if you like an idea, it results from a 'good' program; if you do not, it is the product of a 'mind virus' (McGrath, 2005, p. 125).

We will have more to say about the narrative provided by evolutionary psychology in a later chapter. For now, it is sufficient to point out that there is no empirical evidence to support any of these proposals (including those of Dawkins's mind virus). They make for a nice story, and the ideas perhaps even make some intuitive sense. Evolutionary psychology sees itself as appealing to the scientific theory of evolution for an explanation of all behavior; however, as yet it does not have scientific evidence to support much of what it proposes. This is certainly true for its analysis of ethics and religion. While it is safe to say that some of the practices, beliefs, traditions and so on that form many of the great world religions are human constructions, there is no scientific evidence to support the notion of evolutionary psychology that religion itself is an entirely human enterprise (that is, one that is void of any external or supernatural influence). That issue is, of course, one that is beyond the competency of science to address.

If religion does not have its origin in human experience (that is, is not the result of human initiative), from where might the motivation to worship, a motivation that seems to be virtually universal in the human species, come? Interesting work suggests that our spirituality, if not our religiosity, might be a biological predisposition, not necessarily in the sense of evolutionary psychology, but in the sense that we are born with a need to make attachments, both with other humans and with the 'transcendent'. Research in biology, neuroscience and psychology has led some to suggest that our spirituality just might be innate.

Is Spirituality Innate?

Any discussion of religion needs to consider the question of whether or not religious belief is in fact innate to humans. Given the evidence that in essentially all cultures there is some kind of religious practice, it is reasonable to ask the extent to which the human person is biologically prepared to worship. This is one of the essential questions addressed by the Religious Experience Research Centre, begun by Sir Alister Hardy in 1969, now located at the University of Wales, Lampeter. Alister

Hardy was an Oxford zoologist who became interested in the possibility of a 'biology of the spirit' (Hay, 1990, p. 19). To address this question, Hardy created the above-named center, initially located at Manchester College, Oxford, which was directed by David Hay between 1985 and 1989. The center's aim was to study in a scientific way personal accounts of religious experiences. In so doing, the center collected data on the prevalence of religious experiences among the British population, and found that '... religious or transcendent experience in contemporary Western society ... is widespread and that, in a word, it is normal' (Hay, 1990, p. vii). Hardy and Hay investigated various kinds of experiences. The most common of the categories of experiences studied referred to extraordinary coincidences that suggest there is a pattern unfolding in life. Other reported experiences included a feeling of the presence of God (or a presence not called God), answered prayer, a sacred presence in nature, a preoccupation with the dead (for example, cults of the dead or of ancestors), experiencing that all things are 'one', and a belief in the existence of evil.

David Hay (1990) indicates that as of 1990, almost 50 percent of the population of England claimed to have had these kinds of experiences. Slightly more females than males reported these experiences, but the experiences are associated with a number of positive factors (for example, good mental health, happiness) in both genders (p. 57). Hay also found that people are reluctant to speak of these experiences because of embarrassment and a fear of what others might think, fears he attributes to the influence in England of positivistic science. Hay argues that positivistic science has set the context in which society makes sense of or makes attributions of these experiences, and creates a kind of taboo surrounding religion and spirituality (p. 59). Despite this taboo, however, religious experiences remain common, perhaps because of a biological predisposition. According to Hay, religious awareness is natural to humans. Quoting Hay:

> What has happened in modern industrial cultures such as our own is the loss of a coherent interpretation for this realm of experience, so that it is very poorly integrated into everyday life, with a resulting loss of meaning and value. Nevertheless, as the research work of the Centre has repeatedly shown, the experience is still there, extraordinarily widespread, and, so to speak, in search of understanding. It would seem to me that much of the craziness or extremism associated with modern religious cults is a reaction to the denial of our religiousness. Once our currently tabooed experience of the sacredness of reality is accepted as normal, there is some chance that it can be integrated into, and integrate, our fractured sense of community. (p. 64)

Support for this suggestion comes from a recent report from the Commission on Children at Risk (2003) entitled 'Hardwired to Connect', which addresses why rates of depression, anxiety and conduct disorder have increased in children in the United States over the past twenty years. The cause of this crisis in childhood mental and behavioral health is a 'lack of connectedness ... close connections to other people, and deep connections to moral and spiritual meaning' (p. 5). This commission, composed of over thirty children's doctors, research scientists and mental health professionals from some of the premier universities and research centers in the United States, went on to provide in their report empirical evidence gathered from psychology, neuroscience and other sciences to support their thesis. The commissioners argued that the kind of social institutions that can provide the necessary connectedness have been weakened over the past two decades (institutions such as churches, bowling leagues, card clubs, youth leagues).[1] As a result, there is a growing behavioral and mental health crisis in our children, a crisis played out in the extreme in the tragedy seen at Columbine High School in Colorado, but to a lesser degree in the behavioral problems seen in any elementary classroom today.

The scientific evidence provided in the report points to a basic characteristic of human beings, according to the commissioners. That characteristic is that 'We are hardwired for other people and for moral meaning and openness to the transcendent. Meeting these basic needs for connection is essential to health and to human flourishing' (p. 6). More specifically, the report recommends that we as a society 'pay considerably more attention to young people's moral, spiritual, and religious needs' (p. 7). These are strong words coming from a diverse group of scientists and childhood experts from some of the largest and most highly respected secular institutions in America. The commissioners are not spiritual zealots or religious fundamentalists. They are, however, honestly trying to interpret a vast amount of scientific research that points to the necessity of forming connections with other human beings, and according to the report, with 'the transcendent', however that might be defined. In fairness, the report does not directly address the question of the innateness of spirituality. It is, however, suggestive in that there does seem to be a biological need to form these kinds of connections, some of which might legitimately be considered spiritual in nature. As a result, the report does offer some evidence for the possibility at least that our spirituality, broadly defined perhaps, is biologically based (as Hardy suggested) and innate.

Additional, although indirect, support for an innateness of spirituality and the need to worship the transcendent can be gleaned by examining the rise and fall of atheism in the West. Atheism had its most influential time in history during the eighteenth and nineteenth centuries. Following the French Revolution of 1789, there was great interest in France in the ideas and philosophical positions of atheism, and this interest spread throughout much of Europe. The very idea of atheism became more and more acceptable to the people who shaped the culture of the time, such as philosophers/thinkers La Mettrie, d'Holbach (1723–1789), and the Marquis de Sade (1740–1814). Another individual who contributed to the rise of atheism in Europe, although more accurately a Deist in his personal beliefs, was Voltaire (1694–1778), who wrote satirically and critically about the French Catholic Church. It was during the French Revolutionary period that the notion of an atheistic state was seriously considered, although ultimately rejected (McGrath, 2004a, p. 26).

While atheism did not become official state doctrine in Europe, it did shape the ideas of many intellectuals who would come to influence the culture of twentieth-century Europe and America. Thinkers such as Ludwig Feuerbach (1804–1872), Karl Marx (1818–1883) and Sigmund Freud (1856–1939) had tremendous influence on nineteenth- and twentieth-century economics, politics, medicine and thought. In

1 An excellent account of this weakening of political, civic, social and religious institutions over the latter half of the twentieth century is given in *Bowling Alone: The Collapse and Revival of American Community* by Robert Putnam.

Marx and Freud, both heavily influenced by the philosophy of Feuerbach, we have two clear examples of how an atheistic worldview affected the thinking and writing of these men. For Marx, belief in God was a kind of pacifier (famously called the opium of the people by Marx) for the economic inequities fostered by the market economy of the nineteenth century. Removing the economic inequalities between individuals would make the God belief unnecessary. Thus, the communism that grew out of Marx's writings attempted to expunge belief in God from society and culture. For Freud, belief in God was an illusion based upon wish fulfillment. We believe in God because we want there to be a father-like figure that will protect us. Because there is no God, however, this belief is psychologically unhealthy, and needs to be replaced by beliefs based on the findings of science. The therapeutic technique known as psychoanalysis was developed by Freud to remove these kinds of illusions from the human psyche.

In the twentieth century, many feared that atheism would increasingly replace Christianity and other religions around the world. It was this fear that fueled, at least partially, the Cold War between the United States and the Soviet Union. Instead of atheism becoming more and more accepted by people around the world, however, there has been a resurgence of religion. The case against God fashioned during the eighteenth to mid-twentieth centuries has seemingly stalled, replaced by a growing spirituality, if not outright religiosity, in societies around the world. The belief that there is no God is now recognized as a kind of faith, not a fact that can be 'proved' true by philosophical argument or empirical test. In addition, the trend toward postmodernism that began in the last half of the twentieth century has made a religious worldview just as intellectually viable as a worldview skewed toward atheism. Added to this is the tremendous brutality conducted during the twentieth century by totalitarian regimes in the name of atheism (for example, Stalinism), and one begins to see why we are seeing the twilight of atheism in the world today (McGrath, 2004a). Despite approximately seventy years of state suppression of religion in the former Soviet bloc, faith and religious expression continued in these countries, and was instrumental in the eventual overthrow of communism the world witnessed in the 1980s.

The rise and apparent decline of atheism does not speak directly to the notion of an innate spirituality. However, both the fate of atheism and the scientific findings reported by the Commission on Children at Risk lend indirect support to the possibility of a biological tendency to seek the transcendent and an enduring 'need' to worship and believe in something beyond oneself, even at the risk of losing one's life, as was true in the former Soviet Union. It is, of course, possible that any biological tendency toward the divine is the result of evolutionary mechanisms such as natural selection. It is also, however, just the kind of evidence one would expect to find if we humans were created by God for the purpose of worshiping and having a relationship with him. As C.S. Lewis argued: 'Not only does wishing for something not rule out the existence of the object wished for – it may itself be evidence for its existence' (Armand, 2002, p. 46). That is not, of course, a question that science can answer. It is, however, a reasonable interpretation of some of the evidence that science provides.

What is Religious Experience?

Just as it is difficult to define religion adequately, it is equally problematic to come up with an acceptable definition of religious experience. Behavior, emotion, thought and beliefs can all be considered examples of experiences. Spilka, Hood, Hunsberger and Gorsuch (2003, p. 246) defined religious experience as '… a total way of reacting or being and cannot be reduced to its parts even if such parts could be identified'. In any definition of religious experience, context is crucial, such that if the experience occurs in the context of relating to the transcendent, or in the context of worship, it is considered to be religious experience. A particular pattern of physiological responses (such as increased heart rate, blood pressure and perspiration) might or might not be considered religious depending on where and when the responses occurred. If the responses occurred on a Friday evening at the local high school gymnasium during a basketball game, it would no doubt be considered a nonreligious experience. If the same responses occurred on a Sunday morning during a worship service in church or during private prayer and meditation, they might be interpreted by the person feeling the physiological changes as a religious experience.

Some researchers suggest there is a common core of religious experience that is true across cultures, historical periods and religions. The core of religious experience formulated by Stace includes feelings of the sacred; loss of the sense of self; ineffability (cannot be described in words); feelings of joy, peace and happiness, and a unifying vision in that all things in life are seen to be part of a whole. Other researchers, for example Greeley, also include a loss of concern about worldly problems, heightened emotional intensity, a need to contribute to others, and a certainty that all things will work out for the good (Beit-Hallahmi and Argyle, 1997, pp. 74–6). While the percentage of people reporting these kinds of religious phenomena varies from group to group, the experiences are found in both males and females (females at a higher rate), all ages (frequency generally increasing with age) and across all education levels, social classes and denominational membership (Beit-Hallahmi and Argyle, 1997, pp. 80–81).

William James was particularly interested in extreme religious experience, and today some psychologists, as well as other scientists, study anomalous experiences such as out-of-body and near-death to elucidate the physiological, psychological and social aspects of these rare and highly interesting experiences (Cardena, Lynn and Krippner, 2000). However, less extreme forms of experience can also be considered religious, such as feelings of joy, peace, fear, or even the presence of God or a divinity. Not only are diverse religious experiences studied, they are studied in a variety of different ways using a broad range of methods. Psychologists from a psychoanalytic perspective might be inclined to use case studies to investigate religious experience. Case studies are in-depth investigations of a single individual's behavior, social and historical background, current environmental characteristics and so on. Other psychologists with a more empirical orientation would be more likely to employ correlational or experimental methods to systematically investigate the experience under study. Still others might use interpretative, qualitative and introspective measures to come to a better understanding of the religious phenomenon (Spilka et al., 2003, p. 253).

Despite the belief of some Christians that religion essentially targets the soul or spirit, the body has always been an important factor in religious experience. We use our bodies to worship, so perhaps, as some have suggested, our religious beliefs develop as a result of our physical religious practices. It has also been suggested that our ability to adequately commune with and worship God might be enhanced through teaching our bodies more effective worship behaviors (Coakley, 1997, p. 8). The importance of the body in religious belief and practice can be seen in both Judaism and Christianity. In Judaism, for example, the body is important in Sabbath rituals in the rest given the body on Sabbath, but also in the indulging, rather than neglecting, of the body's needs and appetites. The importance of the body is also seen in death and burial rites intended to make sure the body is not treated in an overly familiar way, but with a high degree of respect (Jacobs, 1997, pp. 78–82).

In Christianity, we also see the importance of physicality in worship. Depending on one's particular denominational preference, believers might face toward the east when reciting the Apostles' Creed, bow at the passing of a cross, kneel during prayer, anoint a body with oil, place hands on another for healing or consecration, or fast during special seasons of the Church year. Clearly, baptism and the Eucharist are sacraments that center on the body (particularly the Eucharist for those of the Catholic faith), and all five senses (vision, hearing, smell, taste, touch) can be stimulated during a worship service. In addition, various meditation practices involve the body through special breathing techniques and bodily postures (Ware, 1997, pp. 102–7). And of course, the Incarnation reminds us that God took the physical, bodily form of a human (Jesus) and came to this physical place (earth) to show us what God is like.

Today, the role of the body in religious experience and expression is increasingly apparent. We are embodied creatures; everything we do and/or experience involves our physical bodies. Chapters 6 and 7 will detail some of the recent evidence from neuroscience and psychology on this concept of embodiment and what it means for religious believers. Here, however, I merely mention that we cannot think about religious experience as involving some nonphysical entity (such as the soul). Our entire body is involved in everything we do, think, feel and believe, and this includes what we do, think, feel and believe about religious matters. At the same time, we must not err by moving from the fact of the body's involvement in religious experience to concluding that religious experience is 'nothing but' the physiological or physical responses of the body. We must not make the mistake of 'reducing' all psychological, social or religious experiences to the physical reactions of which they are comprised. Religious experience is more than physiological reactions in the body; however, those physical responses cannot be ignored or considered unimportant. Our body is involved in all of our experiences. This is no less true for religious experiences.

Religion and Spirituality

If religion is difficult to define, spirituality might be even harder. Many people today consider themselves spiritual, even if they do not think of themselves as being religious. The differences between spirituality and religiosity are often formulated in the following way. Religion, it is thought, tends to be more institutional, formal and authoritarian, whereas spirituality tends to be more subjective, emotional and expressive. Religion tends to be more sociological in nature, whereas spirituality tends to be more psychological. Religion tends to involve beliefs about a deity (although this might not always be the case) and ritualistic behaviors (private or communal), emphasize interest in transcendence and the importance of doctrine, and take place in institutional centers of worship. Spirituality, on the other hand, tends to emphasize personal rather than communal relations with the transcendent, and show less concern with doctrine, beliefs or rituals (Spilka et al., 2003, pp. 9–11). Religion is even thought by some to be 'bad', while spirituality is considered to be 'good'. These supposed distinctions, however, mask the many similarities between these two concepts. Both religion and spirituality take place in a social context, both can be and are interested in the affairs of the individual, and both can be either 'good' or 'bad'. Spirituality and religion are not independent constructs, but are related. The search for the sacred (God, transcendence, the divine, the Ground of Being) is part of religion and spirituality, and is what separates these concepts from other, non-sacred phenomena (Hill and Pargament, 2003).

Measuring Religiosity and Spirituality

When psychology was founded at the end of the nineteenth century, religion and religious experience was a part of the subject matter of the new discipline. Several of the early psychologists recognized that religion was an important element of an individual's life, and believed that any science that attempted to understand human mental experience must consider religion part of the subject matter studied. William James, as mentioned above, was very interested in how religious experience is manifested in human behavior and mental life, as were other major figures in psychology's development (particularly in the United States) such as G. Stanley Hall. Hall trained for the ministry, but changed career directions and became a college professor. He eventually studied the new discipline of psychology under William James at Harvard, becoming the first person to earn a PhD degree with a psychological topic from an American university. After continuing his study of psychology with Wundt in Germany, Hall taught psychology at the first American graduate school in psychology (Johns Hopkins). During the course of his career, Hall founded a number of journals, institutes and laboratories, and was one of the founders of the American Psychological Association, the first professional society for psychology in the United States. Hall was interested in a number of areas in psychology, including child and adolescent psychology, aging and religion.

Hall argued that this new academic or experimental psychology could operate as a kind of 'microscope for the soul' illuminating the inner essence of the human person and helping science to understand the very soul of the individual. He also said that the brain 'is the mouthpiece of God', emphasizing that even using psychology's most naturalistic method of investigation, the study of the brain and nervous system, one was gaining information about the workings not only of man, but of God. Psychology and scripture were compatible, according to Hall, in that the

Bible 'is the great textbook of psychology', providing consistent knowledge with the information being gathered by the scientists trained in the new discipline (Pickren, 2000, p. 1023).

Another figure in psychology's early history was James Angell, professor of psychology and eventually president of the University of Chicago. While a professor at Chicago, Angell mentored John B. Watson, the founder of behaviorism. Angell saw the new psychology as important to religious belief and Christian faith because it would help explain the mysteries of religious life. E.W. Scripture argued that the new psychology could provide a mechanism for building character in children, and that psychology was consistent with religion and was a source of moral blessing (Pickren, 2000, pp. 1023–4).

These psychologists were working during the late nineteenth and early twentieth centuries, and their writings were an attempt to make this new discipline legitimate in the eyes of Americans at the beginning of the twentieth century. These writings were also for a popular audience that was suspicious of the materialism of the new psychology. In trying to gain support for their science, these researchers argued that the new science of psychology would produce results consistent with religious faith, could be used to develop true moral character, and would even provide a basis for true religious discernment.

With the development of psychoanalysis and behaviorism in the early twentieth century (see Chapter 2), interest in religion among psychologists waned. Religion was seen as 'an illusion' and indicator of psychological illness by Freud, and the behaviorist B.F. Skinner wrote that religion was a mechanism of control which claims that the 'power to intervene in the arrangement of reinforcing contingencies [that is, to control behavior] has been vested in it by supernatural authority' (Skinner, 1953, p 352). Religion for much of the middle part of the century was a taboo topic within psychology, and it was during this period that some in the Christian Church became disenchanted with psychology (if they ever thought highly of it in the first place) and began to see psychology as being inconsistent with basic Christian beliefs. In fairness to these believers, psychology could appear to be antireligious in some of its writings, and many psychologists themselves did hold negative views of any kind of knowledge that was not based exclusively on naturalistic assumptions. Psychologists are generally not very religious as individuals, and therefore do not often see the importance of religion in human behavior or mental processing, the very topics psychology is supposed to investigate.

By the end of the twentieth century, however, psychology seemed to have rediscovered religion. Gradually, articles dealing with religion began to appear in the psychological literature. In particular, there was a tremendous rise in the interest among psychologists (as well as physicians, educators and other researchers) in the role of religion (and spirituality) in mental and physical health (see Seybold and Hill, 2001). There was also at this time a growing interest in the psychology of religion that provided a legitimate outlet for the study of religion and its influence on behavior and mental processes. As a reflection of this growing interest, the need for measurements of religion and spirituality became apparent. In order to determine how a construct like religion might affect human behavior, it is necessary to have valid and reliable measures of the variable under investigation, and numerous measures have been constructed during the past thirty-plus years (Hill and Hood, 1999). These measures, totaling over a hundred, reflect the many aspects of spirituality/religiosity, and attempt to assess the cognitive, emotional, interpersonal, behavioral, and even the physiological aspects of the constructs.

Christian Views of Nature and Human Nature

As we have seen, there is great difficulty in trying to define the concepts of religion and spirituality. Psychologists who study religion tend to use operational definitions of religion. How can the concept be measured, for example on a paper-and-pencil test? How would a person who considers himself to be highly religious answer a particular question on a questionnaire? How would a person who considers herself nonreligious answer the same question?

Despite this difficulty, however, a great deal of research is currently being conducted on religion in sociology, psychology, anthropology and related disciplines. One outcome of this research is our understanding that most religions have a view of nature and of human nature. We will begin this section with a discussion of a Christian view of nature itself, and follow that with a look at how Christianity understands human nature. Some of the questions addressed in developing a perspective of nature and of human nature include the following. What is nature? What is nature's relationship to God? What is our proper relationship to nature? Are humans basically good or basically evil? If we humans are fundamentally evil, how did we become that way? For many Christians, the characteristics of both nature itself and human nature are spelled out in the Bible, particularly the early chapters of Genesis (the theologian Emile Brunner suggested, however, that as Christians, we must begin our biblical study of creation in the first chapter of the Gospel of John, where we are told that 'all things were made through him (the Word), and without him was not anything made that was made') (McGrath, 2001, p. 143). These early chapters of Genesis are thought to provide a description of what we are like as human beings, how we became that way, and what the consequences are for our basic nature. But what exactly is a biblical view of nature and of human nature? Is there a definitive position that is clearly spelled out in scripture, or is there instead a range of positions Christians can hold that are biblically supportable?

Considering what the Bible says about nature itself, we begin by trying to define what nature is. John Habgood suggests there are three meanings of the term 'nature'. The first is a specific definition and refers to 'the character or quality of something', and is used to answer questions about what kind of thing a particular object is. The second meaning of the term 'nature' is more general and refers to a directive force. Laws of nature or forces of nature, such as gravitation, would fall under this second meaning of the term. The third use of the term 'nature' is what many people mean when they use the word, and refers to 'the entire physical world' (Habgood, 2002, pp. 3–5).

A biblical view of nature can be understood to have each of these meanings. We can begin in the Old Testament, but must include in our analysis relevant New Testament passages as well. Importantly, the Old Testament tells us that there was a beginning to creation, that God is the creator, that there is order in creation, and that the creation is good. It also emphasizes that God and creation are different. The creation is not made of God and is not God. The New Testament adds to the Old Testament account by telling us that Christ is both the agent of creation and the goal of creation. While the New Testament does not offer a thoroughly worked-out theory of creation, it does provide, in the words of Alister McGrath, 'a series of statements concerning creation which require creation to be viewed in a Christologically focused and Trinitarian manner' (McGrath, 2001, p. 159).

Together, the Old and New Testaments provide what has been termed a Christian doctrine of creation. Fundamental to this doctrine is the belief that God is the creator, that there is order and rationality in the creation, and that humans are part of the creation. While we are part of creation (and therefore separate from the creator), we are also distinguished from the rest of creation by our ability to have a relationship with God. Part of this relationship entails our capacity to grasp something of the created order. According to Aquinas, human rationality corresponds to, but is not identical to, the divine rationality. There is something about the world and the nature of the human mind which allows the patterns and order God put into nature to be seen and understood by us. In doing so, we learn about God, which hopefully furthers the development of our relationship with him. Understanding nature, of course, is the goal of doing science. The sciences are based upon the belief that there is order in the universe. If nature were not orderly, rational and lawful, there would be no point in doing science. The success of the sciences (for example, physics, chemistry, astronomy) testifies to the basic truth of the ordering of nature. So the doctrine of creation provides a plausible and coherent perspective of why there is order in nature and why we can have at least a partial understanding of how nature works.

Regarding a biblical view of human nature, some scientists seem to think that there is only one acceptable view of humanity that is given in the Bible. That view is then critiqued by scientific evidence that is seen as inconsistent with scripture, and the conclusion is reached that the biblical view is incorrect because it is so obviously found in error by what science tells us. Despite making a category mistake by confusing the *methods* of science with the *data* of scripture, these scientists also create a straw man which is easily destroyed. They make the mistaken assumption that the Bible lays out a definitive view of human nature; that view consists of a dualism of body and soul. Their understanding of the biblical picture of humanity consists of the view that God put into a physical body an immaterial soul, and it is this soul or spirit that makes us human. It is this soul that makes us in the image of God. Is this *the* biblical view of human nature? Is this the position that Christians must hold to be consistent with what scripture teaches and to have a high view of the Bible?

As humans, we perceive ourselves to have a body which we believe to be a substance made of matter. With this material body, we can do remarkable things. However, there are some capabilities we possess as humans that are not obviously explicable as bodily functions. For example, it is not immediately clear how thinking, language or consciousness (to mention just three human capabilities) are explained by making reference to our material bodies. These intellectual or mental powers, it appears, are derived from some immaterial substance which many philosophers and theologians have referred to as the soul. This immaterial soul is different from the material body, and the belief that humans have these two substances is known as dualism. (There are different kinds of dualism, and the more specific form of dualism we are talking about here is known as substance dualism, because the adherents to this view hold that humans consist of two different kinds of things or kinds of substances: material substance, the body, and an immaterial substance, the soul. Although these distinctions between dualisms are very important, for the purposes of this discussion we will simply refer to this belief as 'dualism', and not bother with the particular brand of dualism.)

Dualism as a belief about human nature goes back at least as far as the Greek philosopher Plato, who held that there is an eternal soul and a mortal body which are part of an overall dualism of worlds, an eternal world and a temporal world. The eternal soul of a person exists prior to being placed inside a mortal body, and remains trapped there until the body's death. (There is, therefore, in Plato the notion of a universal soul from which an individual soul is a mere shadow.) At the time of death, the soul is freed from the mortal tomb of the body and is able to return to the eternal world from which it originally came. More specifically, Plato believed that there are three aspects of soul: the appetitive, the spirited and the rational. It is the rational aspect of the soul which is possessed by humans and which is eternal. These three types of souls need to be brought under control, and it is the rational soul's job to see that this control is exercised. The rational soul controls the other two aspects much like a charioteer controls the horses that pull a chariot. In order for the soul to function correctly, these three aspects of the soul must work together like the horses must work together to pull a chariot forward. (In the twentieth century, Sigmund Freud used this charioteer imagery to describe the interrelationship between the three structures of the personality, the id, ego and superego. In Freud's vision, the ego must control the id and superego in order for the personality to move forward in a healthy manner.)

Another Greek philosopher, and a student of Plato's, was Aristotle, who broke from his mentor and developed a different conceptualization of the soul. For Aristotle, the concept of 'form' was linked to matter, and the soul is the form of a living thing. All living organisms have souls, because it is the soul that actualizes and directs a living thing, plant, animal or human. The soul is therefore much more closely united with the body in Aristotle's view, and the two cannot easily be separated. Like Plato, Aristotle talked about three kinds of souls, the nutritive soul which provides for growth, reproduction and nutrition; the animal or sensitive soul, found in all animals, which allows for locomotion and basic sensation; and the rational soul only found in humans which enables the intellectual functions such as will, reasoning, knowing.

These themes developed by Greek philosophy influenced the Christian Church via early Church fathers such as Augustine and Aquinas. Augustine based much of his theology and philosophy on a kind of Platonism. To Augustine, the body and soul were easily separated, which was thought to be a necessary condition for belief in life after death. After all, if the soul is not a separate thing from the body, how can humans enjoy eternal life when it is clear that our earthly body dies and returns to dust? In addition, for those Christians who believed in an 'intermediate state' in which the soul rested until the resurrection of the body, the dualism of Plato was considered a requirement. The essence of our personhood, our soul, is a different kind of thing from the body and can exist without the body, either in an intermediate state waiting for the general resurrection, or perhaps in a disembodied form in heaven itself. Either way, Plato's notion of body/soul dualism was appealing to Augustine. Thomas Aquinas took a more Aristotelian view of the soul in which there was greater unity between body and soul. Dualism is still found in Aquinas, however, because of Aquinas's belief in life after death. The dualistic relationship between the body and the soul had the additional benefit of being seen as a kind of model of the relationship between God and humanity (Shults, 2003). Later theologians such as John Calvin (1509–1564) and Martin Luther (1483–1546) also considered the relationship between the body and the soul as crucial to their theologies.

The dualistic view of the relationship between the body and the soul presented above has a long tradition in the Christian Church. Must one hold to the dualistic view to be consistent with the Bible, or can one hold a non-dualistic view of body and soul and still be faithful to scripture? Is the received view of how the body and soul relate (dualism) even biblical, or has it been too much influenced by Greek philosophy? Is it instead the case that a different view of human nature, one that does not see the body and the soul as being two different kinds of things, is more true to scripture?

This is exactly the case being made by numerous biblical scholars, including those considered to be evangelical in their theological orientation. Their position is that a more holistic view of humans, one in which the body and the soul are not distinct substances but are united, is the correct biblical view of human nature: 'In the last two centuries, biblical scholars have increasingly moved toward a consensus that both the Hebrew Bible and the New Testament provide a holistic model of the human person' (Shults, 2003, p. 175). What is the evidence for this holistic vision of personhood?

Obviously, the words used in a particular language are crucial in conveying the message the writer or speaker wishes to send. As the message is translated from one language to another, it can be altered because of the choice of words used in the translation. When we read the Bible, we must keep in mind that the original language of scripture was not what we read today. The writers of the New Testament used Greek when they wrote; the writers of the Old Testament used Hebrew. Much of the Old Testament, however, comes to us in written form after being conveyed verbally from one generation to the next. So, in order to begin to determine what the Old Testament or the New Testament has to say about human nature, we need to look at what the significant Hebrew and Greek words are and how they were understood by the writers and readers (or hearers) of the original culture.

In the Old Testament, there are a number of words that are used when making reference to human nature. For example, the word *nephesh* (meaning 'throat' or 'neck') is often translated as 'soul' or 'life'. Another word used in this context is *basar*, which means 'flesh' and 'embodiedness', and is sometimes used to refer to kinship relationships (for example, Genesis 37:27). The Hebrew word *leb* means 'heart' or the 'center of activity of the self', and *ruach* is often translated as 'person', 'breath' or 'spirit'. Each of these words can be used to refer to that aspect of our existence we call soul, self or spirit, and suggests the notion of the unity of the person. Each term indicates wholeness, not division, and implies that we are not bodies with souls (or bodies with souls and spirits), but are unified persons. We are, in other words, embodied souls. A key scripture passage in this regard is Genesis 2:7, which reads (in the Revised Standard Version): 'then the Lord God formed man of dust from the ground, and breathed into his nostrils the breath of life; and man became a living being [*nephesh*]'. Here, the word *nephesh* is translated as 'soul' in the King James Version of the Bible, as being in the RSV, and as 'person' in the New Living Translation (Stone, 2004, p. 53).

In the New Testament, Greek words for heart, spirit, body, soul are all used to refer to the whole person (Shults, 2003, p. 175). *Pneuma* means 'spirit' in Greek, and *psychē* is translated as 'soul', but these words are used in ways that, like the Hebrew Old Testament words, suggests a unity and holism. Other Greek words typically used in the context of the person are *kardia* (2 Corinthians 3:14–16, 2:4, 7:3) and *nous* (Romans 12:1), which also refer to the whole person. *Soma* (which means 'body' in Greek) is used to refer to humans as embodied persons. The body is the person, and Paul in 1 Corinthians emphasizes the resurrection of the body, the whole being or person. In Romans 8:19–23, the terms 'flesh' (*sarx*) and 'spirit' (*pneuma*) do not suggest a dualism of substances. Living in the spirit suggests a person whose whole being is oriented toward the spirit; the fleshly person one whose whole being is oriented toward earthly, fleshly desires (Shults, 2003, p. 178).

The scriptures, these biblical scholars tell us, depict the human person as a whole, a unity, not as a material body with an immaterial soul or spirit. These various terms (such as body, soul, spirit, heart, mind) are different *perspectives* one can bring when looking at the individual, not different substances. As Shults puts it, the Bible is concerned with the whole person, particularly the salvation of the whole person (p. 178). Dualism, these scholars suggest, comes not from the Bible, but from Greek philosophers such as Plato, whose influence on the early Church contributed to a mistranslation of the original New Testament manuscripts. Instead of understanding *psychē*, for example, as a holistic term for 'personhood', the term was misinterpreted (under the influence of Plato's philosophy) to mean a 'disembodied, immaterial and immortal soul'. This understanding was consistent with Greek philosophy (for example, Platonism), but not with the intended meaning of the original scriptural passage.

Is the Alternative to Dualism Monism?

Some are rightly concerned that the alternative to a dualistic vision of the human person is pure materialism. If we are not *both* a physical body and an immaterial soul, then we must be *merely* a physical body. This view of personhood as a singular kind of thing (for example, body) is known as monism, and is often, correctly, equated with a materialistic philosophy that believes that matter is all that exists. It is partly for this reason that some theologians (such as John Cooper) still hold to dualism as the correct view of human nature, despite the evidence cited above that the Bible does not teach dualism (Cooper, 2001, p. 219). Dualism is thought to be necessary for life after death and the intermediate state; the monistic alternative of human nature is not considered compatible by these theologians with belief in an afterlife. The alternative to dualism is not necessarily materialistic monism, however. Biblical scholars suggest that a proper reading of scripture (both Old and New Testaments) leads one to conclude that belief in a distinct, immaterial soul is not necessary for the continuation of personhood after death, either in an intermediate state or at an immediate resurrection (Gutenson, 2004, p. 132). The Bible teaches the resurrection of the whole person, a re-embodiment, and eternal life, not the existence of a disembodied soul after death of the body (Green, 2004b, p. 100; Peters, 1999, p. 323). The important point for our purpose is that the biblical portrait of the person as a unity and a whole is consistent with the growing literature coming from neuroscience and psychology which we will review in later chapters. That scientific literature also suggests that the human person is not composed of a physical thing and an immaterial thing (or substance). The neuroscientific and psychological research we will consider indicates that the human person is a physical creature, and that the mental functions and capabilities that used to be attributed to an immaterial soul can be understood to be the result of physical forces. Far from evoking resistance from believers, these findings can be welcomed because they coincide with the biblical literature and remind us that we are indeed 'fearfully and wonderfully made'.

Chapter 4

Philosophy of Science

When most people think of a psychologist, they think of a person sitting in an office listening to another person, perhaps reclined on a couch, talk about their problems. If that is the first image one has of a psychologist, perhaps the second would be of a white-coated scientist watching a rat running through a maze or pressing a bar for food. It is that second image that is created when one thinks of B.F. Skinner. Burrhus Frederic Skinner (1904–1990) graduated from college as an English major, but studied psychology in graduate school, eventually obtaining his PhD in psychology from Harvard University. Skinner believed, as did many others during the middle portion of the twentieth century, that a purely scientific study of behavior was not only possible, but necessary in order for psychology to make the kind of progress seen in other disciplines such as physics and physiology. He spent much of his academic life studying the behavior of rats and pigeons in 'Skinner boxes', enclosed cages where the animal can be trained to make a particular response (for example, pressing a lever for a rat or pecking a disk or 'key' for a pigeon) and observed to see how that behavior can be modified based on what happens after the response is made. This kind of psychology is known as operant psychology, and Skinner was, before his death in 1990, perhaps the best-known psychologist in history. His book *Walden Two* was a fictional account of how his operant psychology principles could be applied broadly to produce a utopian society. Skinner was a behaviorist (that is, a psychologist who believes the proper subject matter for psychology is behavior, not mental processes), who remained consistent in his views while others around him became increasingly cognitive or mentalistic in their approach to psychology. He argued that all behavior, even thought, which he considered subvocal behavior, could be studied using the methodology of the natural sciences. Skinner believed that science has a number of characteristics that clearly separate it from other approaches to knowledge. It might even be said that Skinner believed that science was the only legitimate method to obtain knowledge, and that the only truth that exists is scientific truth. In this regard, Skinner followed a positivist view of how to practice science.

Positivism is a philosophy of science which sees science as a purely objective enterprise. The scientist is completely independent of the subject being investigated. The scientist conducting an experiment merely observes what happens; the scientist is a collector of data, and these data are unaffected by the person observing them. After collecting the data, the scientist then analyzes and interprets the results, and arrives at some conclusion. This entire process, however, is completely objective and unaffected by the beliefs, opinions or expectations of the individual scientist. Science is a sterile process of data collection and analysis. Substitute one scientist for another and you will get the same set of data and the same conclusions about what those data mean.

This positivistic philosophy of what science is and how the work of science is conducted greatly influenced not only Skinner, but other psychologists as well. Since its founding in 1879, psychology has wanted to be like the natural sciences of physics and physiology. By the 1930s, behaviorism was a dominant approach to psychology, and while there were differences among the behaviorists in their views of what psychology is and how psychological research should be conducted, a positivistic philosophy of science was accepted by many, which resulted in a natural science approach to the study of behavior. The positivistic approach to science, however, was challenged in the latter half of the twentieth century by those who argued that science is not a purely objective and sterile enterprise. This new philosophy of science is known as postpositivism, and it proposes that the data scientists collect are 'theory-laden' – that is to say, observations and the data derived from them are not purely objective. A scientist comes to the laboratory experiment with certain beliefs about what will be observed, about what constitutes data, and about how those predicted observations might be interpreted. Thus it is not completely accurate, so postpositivism argues, to say that a scientific theory emerges out of objectively observed data. Instead, it is more accurate to say that the theory which the scientist is testing helps to identify what the data are.

Postpositivism

The challenges to positivism as a philosophy of science are clearly laid out in the book *The Structure of Scientific Revolutions* by Thomas Kuhn (1970). In this important work, Kuhn argues that all scientists hold a particular worldview, or paradigm, which consists of assumptions about how the world works and how science must be practiced. These paradigms must be held for science to successfully solve the puzzles of nature. Occasionally, however, these scientific worldviews are challenged by data that do not fit into the accepted paradigm. If these challenges are not resolved within the existing paradigm, a new paradigm might emerge and replace the old. When this happens, a scientific revolution occurs, according to Kuhn. An example of such a scientific revolution is the replacement of a geocentric view of the solar system with Copernicus's (1473–1543) sun-centered paradigm. Gradually during the seventeenth century, more and more astronomers (for example, Galileo) came to accept the truth of Copernicus's approach, and the new paradigm eventually replaced the old. The new paradigm came to influence how the astronomers of the day understood the arrangements of the planets, the sun, and importantly, the earth. The new paradigm also made certain predictions about the movement of these celestial bodies, and was more aesthetically pleasing and simpler than the old earth-centered model, which had become more and more complex and cumbersome. Kuhn in his book argues that science progresses through the removal of old paradigms and the introduction of new ones.

During the revolution, however, the differing paradigms compete for acceptance. The old paradigm tries to maintain its role, and the new approach tries to get scientists to jump ship from the old worldview to the new perspective proposed by the novel paradigm. As Kuhn argues, this competition between paradigms is not resolved by 'proofs'. The proponents of the two paradigms often differ on whether there is even a problem with the old model. If it is agreed that problems with the old paradigm exist, it is not always clear that the new paradigm will be able to solve the problems any better than the old. The switch, therefore, from the old paradigm to the new is more like a conversion experience than a step-by-step logical reasoning process. Kuhn says that the decision to switch from the old paradigm to the new 'can only be made on faith' that the new paradigm will outperform the old (Kuhn, 1970, p. 158).

The postpositivistic approach suggests that there is a social nature to science. Theories arise, in part, from the creative acts of scientists and from the society in which these scientists work. In addition, both the observer (the scientist) and the object being observed form a kind of relationship during the course of a scientific experiment. Work in physics suggests that observing an electron actually changes the behavior of the electron, and certainly watching human behavior in a psychology experiment (or in everyday experience) can change the behavior of the person being observed. If we know we are being watched, we behave differently than if we believe our behavior is not being observed. Philosopher of science Michael Polanyi talks about 'personal knowledge' and how there is personal participation of the knower in all knowledge (Polanyi, 1958). As we assess evidence, even scientific evidence, Polanyi suggests we are engaging in an act of discretionary judgment. This approach to understanding data as an inherently subjective process is vastly different from how positivistic science views the interpretation of collected scientific evidence as objective and independent of the observer. Positivistic science sees data as describable in a theory-free language, but postpositivism suggests that there are no theory-free data. The theory (Kuhn would say paradigm) determines, in part at least, the phenomena studied by science, the form of the question asked by the scientist, and the choice of how to measure the object under study. Science, in short, is not purely objective, but has subjectivism embedded throughout the process.

Postpositivism has now replaced positivism as the accepted philosophy of how science is conducted. Given this change in approach, some see a closer connection between science and theology. It is not argued by these individuals that science and theology are doing the same kind of work, it is rather suggested that there is greater overlap between postpositivistic science and theology than is seen between theology and positivistic science. For example, Jones (1994) maintains that the parallels between postpositivistic science and religion include similarities in subject matter. Both science and religion are concerned with real aspects of human experience. The particular components of human experience may differ, but human experience is studied by science and religion, and the 'findings' of both must be consistent with what people know to be true in their lives. Second, both scientific theories and religious doctrines must be coherent: that is to say, both should be consistent with other accepted theories or doctrines. What one believes about the nature of Jesus Christ must be coherent or consistent with what one believes about the nature of the Trinity. Theological doctrines must be interconnected: they must go together in a meaningful way. The same is true of scientific theories. They should also be interconnected, hopefully in an elegant and simple manner. For example, the same theory that predicts the movement of the planet Mars should also predict the movement of Venus. If it does not, it is not considered a good scientific theory. Third, both scientific theories and religious doctrines are held provisionally. Scientific theories are never 'proven' beyond all doubt. Conclusions in science are always incomplete, tentative and subject to revision based on new evidence. This is not to say that scientific theories are mere opinion. Science provides reliable methods for testing and evaluating theories, and established theories have substantial evidence to support them. It is to say, however, that science does not lead to absolute certainty. In a similar way, religious doctrines can be and have been revised based on new 'evidence'. One only has to look at the Protestant Reformation to see examples of theological doctrines that were modified based on new interpretations of personal experience. Finally, both scientific theory and religious doctrine can elicit strong, even passionate, devotion. While there are many differences between science (even postpositivistic science) and religion, both are rational, social attempts to understand a part of reality, are shaped by fundamental assumptions, and are accountable to human experience (Jones, 1994, p. 190).

Realism in Science

The notion that science is a social enterprise leads some to argue that scientific knowledge itself is a social construction: that the objects and events about which information is acquired through scientific research do not exist independently of that research. This antirealism view is addressed by Roy Bhaskar (1997), who argues for critical realism in science. Bhaskar recognizes that scientific knowledge is, in part, socially and historically determined. For example, what we currently know about the neural mechanisms and functioning of the human mind is limited by the available technology in the early twenty-first century (for example, brain imaging technologies such as fMRI and PET scans). Nevertheless, Bhaskar maintains that the neural events themselves that make up mental experience exist independently of our knowing about them. Mind, therefore, is not a socially constructed phenomenon, even though what we know about the mind is a function, in part, of our cultural and historical place. In other words, what really exists (ontology in philosophical terminology) is not determined by or limited to what can be observed (methodology). This error, known by philosophers as the epistemic fallacy, was a major mistake made by many positivists who defined reality in terms of what they could observe. In opposition to this, critical realism sees the world as stratified in its mechanisms, meaning that there is 'an ordered series of generative mechanisms', in which the lower mechanisms representing physics and chemistry can explain the higher mechanisms (for example, biological and psychological) without explaining them away or replacing them (Collier, 1994, p. 48).

Because nature is stratified in this way, science too must be stratified in its methods. Science is divided or stratified into distinct kinds. One model of this stratification of the sciences is to consider the various disciplines that make up science as existing in a pyramid, with physics forming the base (as shown in Figure 4.1). (When the term 'science' is used in this fashion it is not limited to the natural or even the behavioral or social sciences. 'Science' in this model refers to knowledge, which is the original meaning of the term. *Scientia,* from which the English word 'science' is derived, is Latin for knowledge of any kind.)

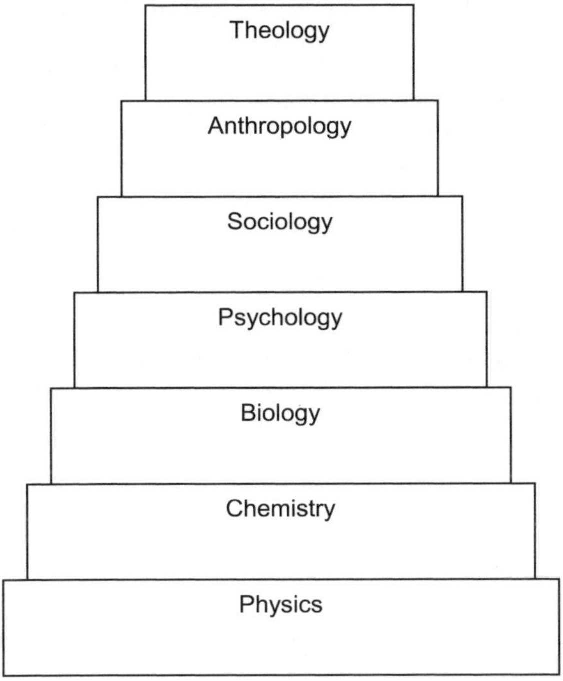

Figure 4.1 A stratified model of the sciences.

Physics, therefore, is considered a foundational science. Above physics is chemistry, and above chemistry is biology. As we move higher on the pyramid, we find the sciences of psychology, sociology, anthropology, with perhaps theology at the top. (This list includes just a few of the disciplines that study the various strata of reality.) Sciences at the bottom of the pyramid are more basic than those near the top. Physics, therefore, is more basic than chemistry, which is more basic than biology, which is more basic than psychology, and so on. Being more basic, however, does not mean that a science at a higher level can be replaced by a science at a lower level. The mechanisms studied and uncovered by psychology are not replaced by or reduced to the mechanisms described by biology. The mechanisms at both levels are irreducible. Knowledge of behavior and mental processes obtained using the methods of psychology is not reducible to nor replaced by knowledge of neurophysiology obtained using the methods of biology. Both psychology and biology provide true knowledge and use legitimate methods, given the stratum investigated. The positivistic notion that all psychology can be reduced to biology, and all biology to chemistry, and all chemistry, ultimately, to physics simply does not reflect the stratification of nature and of reality.

Phenomena at the higher strata will be governed by more than one kind of law, so more than one kind of method is required to understand the phenomena. The goal of science in general is to dig deeper and deeper into the strata of reality to uncover the mechanisms at work at the more basic levels. In this regard, science is never finished in its work. As soon as a deeper or lower-level mechanism is uncovered (for example, a chemical mechanism for schizophrenia), a still deeper mechanism awaits discovery (for example, the physics of neurotransmitter transport). Just as the quality of wetness emerges out of the proper combination of hydrogen and oxygen, so too the higher-level laws are said to emerge out of or to be rooted in the lower. Because they emerge out of the lower, the higher-level mechanisms cannot be reduced to or be replaced by the lower, and we can never predict or completely understand the higher-level mechanisms from our knowledge of the lower (Collier, 1994, p. 110). Just as we can not predict the wetness of water by our knowledge of the properties of hydrogen and oxygen individually, consciousness (a high-level phenomenon studied by psychology) cannot be thoroughly explained or anticipated by an understanding of neurochemistry or neurophysiology, even though these lower-level mechanisms might be very helpful in providing some important information about the nature of conscious experience. Each stratum is real and requires study using the methods appropriate for that level. It is reality and existence (ontology) that determines correct methodology (epistemology), not, as the positivists would have it, epistemology which determines what is real.

The Role of Naturalism and Reductionism in Psychology and Neuroscience

Today, the word 'science' no longer refers, as it did in the original Latin, to knowledge of any kind. For the last 300 years, science increasingly has come to mean a particular kind of knowledge which derives from studying nature and the physical world. In addition, science now means the search for naturalistic mechanisms that can explain the operations of the natural and physical world. Two philosophical assumptions that science has adopted are naturalism and materialism. Naturalism is the belief that natural (as opposed to supernatural) mechanisms explain how the physical universe operates. A ball falls to the ground when released not because of a supernatural force, but because of the natural process of gravity. A plane takes off, flies at 30 000 feet and lands safely because of natural processes, not because of any supernatural activity. Science as it is currently practiced and defined (at least by the vast majority of scientists) looks for these natural mechanisms and is incapable of discovering any processes outside of these natural ones. Science is limited to the search for natural mechanisms and laws. This limitation is known as methodological naturalism, and is a fundamental position held among natural, behavioral and social scientists. As mentioned above, reality is stratified, and each level or stratum requires its own methods. Methodological naturalism might not be appropriate for investigation into some levels of reality (for example, the theological level), but it is appropriate for investigation into the more basic levels such as physics, chemistry and biology. Some people become concerned, however, when methodological naturalism is applied to the study of phenomena in the psychological stratum of reality.

Another belief held by the vast majority of scientists is methodological reductionism, which means that as a scientist, it is perfectly appropriate and even necessary to reduce the phenomenon you are studying to its more fundamental elements. For example, if a mechanic wanted to know how an engine worked, that mechanic might tear the engine apart (reduce it to its more fundamental level) and see how the individual parts operate. Then, that mechanic might begin the process of putting the parts back together, and when that was done, a good understanding of how the engine (as a whole) functions would be gained. A scientist in the lab typically follows a similar kind of process. If one wants to know how a particular phenomenon in nature works, one might break that phenomenon down into its component parts and study the parts individually. Then, after the individual parts are understood, they can be recombined and a better understanding of the whole phenomenon is obtained. For example, if a psychologist wanted to know about schizophrenia (a severe disorder that affects a person's thinking, perception and emotional responses), they could 'reduce' the disorder to abnormalities within the brain (for example, chemical imbalances, brain cell loss), and study it at that level. This is a perfectly reasonable and effective way of learning more about the natural mechanisms involved in this very destructive and debilitating disorder.

A mistake would be made, however, if the psychologist reducing schizophrenia to the underlying neurological abnormality assumes that schizophrenia is 'nothing but' a brain disorder. There are other levels at which schizophrenia can be studied, including the effect of the disorder on an individual's psychological life, social life and spiritual life. One can also study the effects of schizophrenia on the victim's family and friends, or how society as a whole is affected by the disorder through the loss of productivity in those who suffer from the disease and in the cost of treating the illness. The phenomenon of schizophrenia is stratified (as is all reality), and can be studied using different methodologies, some of which look for naturalistic mechanisms, others of which do not.

The natural sciences (physics, chemistry, biology and some areas of psychology) use methodological reductionism to study those levels of reality (for example, disorders such as schizophrenia) where natural mechanisms (such as chemical imbalances and brain damage) are at work. This does not mean that other, nonnatural mechanisms are not also implicated; it is simply to say that if nonnatural mechanisms are involved, they will not be detected by the natural sciences. Adopting methodological naturalism and reductionism are necessary positions for scientists to hold when they are working in a lab or in the field, but they can hold these beliefs without also assuming that natural mechanisms are all that exist (ontological naturalism) or that reality is nothing more than the reduced individual parts that make up some phenomenon. A psychologist can use methodological reductionism to study some mental or behavioral process, for example the brain areas involved in empathy and forgiveness, without assuming that empathy and forgiveness are nothing more than patterns of neural activity. And a psychologist might also study the natural brain mechanisms involved in religious experience without believing that religious experience is nothing but a natural process devoid of any supernatural activity. The critical realism of Bhaskar and others recognizes that because reality is stratified and multileveled, many methods are required to study reality. The nature of the phenomena at a given level of reality determines which method is most appropriate. Investigating phenomena at the psychological level using methodological naturalism and reductionism does not preclude the study of emergent phenomena using additional methods or studying higher strata of reality using methods more appropriate to those levels. Various methods are needed to adequately understand the multileveled nature of reality of which both God and his creation are a part.

Chapter 5

Integration Issues

For some people, science is best represented by a person such as Richard Dawkins, Charles Simonyi Professor of the Public Understanding of Science at the University of Oxford. Dawkins is famous as a leading zoologist and proponent of Darwinian evolution. He is also well known as an ardent atheist, ready to attack religion and faith at any opportunity. Dawkins regards faith as one of the world's great evils, on a par with smallpox, HIV and other viruses that need to be eradicated (McGrath, 2005, p. 84). He sees belief in God as similar to belief in the tooth fairy and unicorns. Religion is dangerous, faith a cop-out. Science and religion are incompatible, just like science and magic are incompatible. Science, to Dawkins, requires atheism, and while perhaps one could have logically been an atheist before Darwin, after Darwin a scientist must be an intellectually fulfilled atheist.

Dawkins is an eminent and widely known scientist; his personal 'beliefs' about faith and religion, however, are certainly not required opinions for a scientist to hold. There are many scientists who find no incompatibility between their religious beliefs and their work as a scientist. One example of such a person is John Stapylton Habgood, a physiologist and pharmacologist who was also Archbishop of York before his retirement in 1995 (Seybold, 2005). Another is Alister McGrath, Professor of Historical Theology at Oxford University, who is not only a highly regarded and widely known theologian, but who also has a doctorate in biophysics. One could name others from Great Britain, the United States, Canada, Australia, Germany, Russia and many other nations who have made substantial contributions in their respective scientific disciplines and who also have written extensively in theology or how their disciplines relate to their religious beliefs. Noted examples include John Polkinghorne (mathematical physics); Arthur Peacocke (physical biochemistry); Henry Schaefer (chemistry); and Fraser Watts, Malcolm Jeeves, David Myers and Warren Brown (psychology and neuroscience), to mention just a few. In addition, while they may not have written books or scholarly articles on theology, there are innumerable scientists who are practicing Christians or who are believers in other religious traditions (for example, Judaism or Islam). Francis Collins, for example, is the Director of the National Human Genome Research Institute in the United States. Collins, an evangelical Christian and one of the world's foremost geneticists, sees 'no conflict in what the Bible tells me about God and what science tells me about nature'. For Collins, 'scientific discovery is also an occasion of worship' (Van Biema, 2005, p. 34).

These examples serve to illustrate that the position taken by Dawkins (and to greater or lesser extent scientists such as Steven Pinker, psychologist at Harvard University, Daniel Dennett, Professor of Philosophy and Director of the Center for

Cognitive Studies at Tufts University, and the late Francis Crick, co-discoverer of the structure of DNA) is not required of a scientist. As John Habgood puts it:

> There is no need for science and Christianity to be in fundamental conflict. But in an age when conflicts lie not very far in the past … there are bound to be tensions. … such tensions do not necessarily imply that one side is right and the other wrong. On the contrary, it is possible to be both an honest Christian and an honest scientist, and to find the two allegiances both illuminating and correcting one another. (Habgood, 1964, p. 151)

The position on science and religion held by Dawkins, Pinker, Dennett and others is thought by many to be how scientists have always viewed religion – with suspicion. (This view is even seen in some popular writings, for example the plot of the novel *Angels and Demons* by best-selling author Dan Brown revolves around a battle between open and honest science and the secretive and oppressive Catholic Church.) In the late nineteenth century, two books were published that presented such a historical view of science and religion (Draper, 1874; White, 1896). The thesis put forth by these authors saw science and religion at war with each other for ultimate authority within society. Science is seen as a rational process that seeks to uncover truth within the universe. Religion is viewed as an irrational process that is based on faith and superstition – an enterprise that cannot find truth because it is not seeking or looking for anything that is real. In the Draper-White thesis, science and reason ultimately triumph over religion as the source of authority and knowledge.

This warfare and conflict position, however, is no longer held by those who have seriously studied the relationship between science and religion. A more diverse and complex view of the relationship between science and religion is needed, and has been provided by historians such as John Hedley Brooke, Professor of Science and Religion at the University of Oxford (Brooke, 1991). Such a complex position sees the relationship between religion and science as a function of local conditions existing at a particular time and place. Yes, the Church has at times seemed to be at odds with science. The Galileo Affair, the church's response to Darwin, and the Scopes trial are often used as examples of the conflict between religion and science. Looking at the history of science and religion, however, reveals that these 'typical' interactions between people of science and people of faith are anything but typical or usual. Historically, science and religion can be understood as mutually benefiting each other, and what we think we know about the Galileo Affair, the response of the Church to Darwin, and the trial of John Scopes is often mistaken. More often than not throughout history, science and religion have gotten along quite well. Moreover, while there was certainly a type of science practiced in Islamic counties and in the Middle and Far East, early modern science emerged, to a great extent, from a Western European culture heavily infused with Judeo-Christian principles and way of life (Grant, 1996, pp. 171–91).

This chapter will review some of the history of how science and religion have interacted. By reviewing this history, we will get an idea of what historians mean when they say that the relationship between religion and science is complex. We will take a brief look at what we know about some of the major 'conflicts' between religion and science in the past, and see whether received knowledge about these incidents matches what actually occurred. We will also consider four models of how science and religion might go together (Barbour, 1990, 1997). These models are provided by Ian Barbour, the man some say created the contemporary study of science and religion. By studying these four approaches to how science and religion might 'go together', we can begin to see the diversity and complexity of the subject with which we are dealing.

Science and Religion in History

Any attempt to discuss the relationship between science and religion must begin by recognizing the difficulty of defining the terms. Religion is widely recognized as being hard to define (see Chapter 3). Some suggest that the term should no longer be used at all because it is so difficult for people from diverse backgrounds to agree about what it means. Others, however, argue that the word religion is still a useful term that is used to distinguish certain beliefs and practices from those described as art, science or some other kind of human experience (Ward, 2004, p. 24). If we begin by considering religion as belief in a supernatural being or a commitment to some transcendent 'other' and include organized institutions with creeds, rituals, moral imperatives, propositional claims and so on, all conforming to a rationalist orientation to truth, we will come close to a 'common' understanding of what has passed for religion since the seventeenth century (Harrison, 2006). As in previous chapters of this book, we will limit ourselves to a discussion of how science relates to the religion of Christianity.

Science also has numerous definitions. Originally used to mean 'knowledge', the definition of science now encompasses both content and methodology. For most people, science refers specifically to the natural sciences of physics, chemistry, biology and related disciplines, and is barely a century old (Harrison, 2006). A broader understanding of science might also include psychology in that list. Scientists of the past (for example, Newton) considered themselves natural philosophers, and the concerns of religion and 'science' were fully integrated. Because modern definitions of science and religion are different from how they were used in the past, it is difficult to consider how the two have related throughout history. Following historians such as Brooke, however, we are sensitized to the notion that we should avoid simple approaches to science and religion, recognizing their complex relationship, one shaped by specific events and concerns of place and time.

For proponents of the warfare thesis, religion and science are now and have always been in conflict. One must ultimately choose between pursuing truth and knowledge using empirical, scientific methods (the only legitimate approach), and resorting to the backward, irrational and superstitious approach favored by religion. This conflict view is supposedly supported by the many examples of progressive science being suppressed by the established Church. As mentioned above, this does not represent an accurate portrait of how science and religion have related throughout history. Isaac Newton, Francis Bacon, René Descartes, Robert Boyle were Christians who were instrumental in the development of modern science during the Renaissance. Nevertheless, proponents of this conflict thesis attempt to support their view by recalling the suppression of Galileo as he tried to convince Church authorities of the truth, supposedly well established by science at the time, of the heliocentric theory of the solar system. A second argument for the constant warfare between Church and science is the reception of Darwinism by ecclesiastical authorities. This negative reaction is best typified, so the reasoning goes, by the famous debate between Sam Wilberforce, the Bishop of Oxford, and Darwin's bulldog, Thomas Huxley. A final piece of evidence provided is the so-called Monkey Trial of John Scopes in Dayton, Tennessee, in 1925. Scopes, according to legend, was taken from his classroom by town authorities and the police, and arrested for teaching evolution to high school students in violation of state law. Once again, progressive science was suppressed by the backward-looking state laws that were based upon a literalist biblical account of creation, particularly the creation of man. Unfortunately for the conflict thesis, much of what is commonly known about the Galileo Affair, the Wilberforce-Huxley debate, and the Scopes trial is legend and myth, sprinkled with some fact. When these historical events are studied in depth by historians, a more complicated picture of these incidents emerges, a picture that does not indicate as much 'conflict' has many suppose.

The Galileo Affair is perhaps the best-known example of supposed suppression of science by religion (the Catholic Church in particular), and is considered (inaccurately) a classic case of Church ignorance and authority over scientific truth and reason. Galileo was an advocate of Copernicus's theory (heliocentrism) that the sun is the center of the solar system, and that the planets, including the earth, travel around the sun. This theory was in disagreement with the geocentric theory, which had the earth as the center of the solar system with all the planets, the moon and the sun revolving around it. According to the story, Galileo published indisputable evidence in favor of heliocentrism, but was forced to recant his belief under threat of torture and death at the hands of Church authorities who believed that the Bible taught that the sun revolved around the earth. After all, Joshua commanded the sun to stop its movement across the sky (Joshua 10:12–13), and other scripture passages support the fixed position of the earth (for example, Psalm 93:1). The picture painted is one of Galileo and scientific evidence on one side, and Church tradition, superstition and the Bible on the other. This is the image created in most productions of the play *The Life of Galileo* by Bertolt Brecht.

In reality, however, the Galileo Affair is a complex interplay of historical events in the Catholic Church (for example, the Counter-Reformation), legal issues and exegetical standards (for example, the Council of Trent declaring that only the Pope and bishops can interpret the Bible). The Galileo Affair was more than a simple conflict between science and religion; it had personal and political dimensions as well (Lindberg, 2003). The outcome was heavily influenced by local circumstances existing in Rome as well as in Florence and Pisa, Galileo's home bases, by personality differences between Galileo and other significant figures in the affair (Galileo was famously abrasive and arrogant), and importantly, by differences regarding how cosmological claims were to be resolved, via reference to biblical revelation, evidence of the senses and reason, or some combination. The Galileo Affair was as much a conflict within the Church over these issues as it was a conflict between the Church and science. All of the major figures in the incidents leading up to Galileo's trial in 1633, including Galileo himself, believed in the authority of the Bible, and many of them, including most of the Church authorities, were natural philosophers. The Church did ultimately decide against Galileo. The majority of the scientists of the day, however, also thought that the geocentric theory was correct. Galileo was not only opposed in his heliocentrism by the Church, he was opposed by accepted science as well. The Church did not reject science in favor of biblical revelation, the Church accepted what the science of the day believed (that is, that the sun did, in fact, revolve around the earth). Contrary to what he maintained, Galileo, in the opinion of both the Church authorities and the scientists of the day, had not demonstrated or proved that the heliocentric theory was true and correct. The position taken by Galileo's judges (that Galileo had not convincingly shown that heliocentrism was better science than geocentrism) was in step with the majority scientific opinion. His recantation was not under threat of torture or death, but he did spend the remainder of his life (nine years) under house arrest in his villa outside Florence. During these years, Galileo wrote some of his most well-known work.

The second famous example of 'conflict' between science and religion was the debate on Darwin's evolutionary theory between Samuel Wilberforce and Thomas Huxley that took place at the meeting of the British Association for the Advancement of Science held in Oxford in June of 1860. Wilberforce was the Bishop of Oxford, and Huxley was an ardent supporter of evolutionary theory and friend of Charles Darwin. According to the story, Wilberforce and Huxley were debating when Wilberforce tried to belittle Huxley and evolutionary theory by asking him (Huxley) if he thought he had descended from apes on his mother or his father's side of the family. Huxley supposedly then responded by saying he would rather be related to an ape than to a bishop. The crowd roared its approval; one woman went into a Victorian swoon as a result of the exchange between the two men and the Bishop's clear humiliating defeat at the hands of the scientist. Huxley had delivered a tremendous blow for Darwinism against the stagnant and backward views of Church dogma. It was seen as a defining moment in science–religion relations. Again, science had won the day.

Just like with the Galileo Affair, however, there is some question as to the truth of the story of the Wilberforce–Huxley debate. How much of the story is accurate and how much is legend made up after the fact to make Huxley (and science) look good and Wilberforce (and by extension religion) look bad? Contemporary accounts of the debate do not indicate that Huxley had delivered a serious blow to Wilberforce. They instead indicate that both gentlemen represented their positions well. Some accounts of the meeting do not even mention the Wilberforce–Huxley exchange, instead reporting on the other scholars who spoke that day. The event does not seem to have left any lasting impressions on the attendees, and the importance of the debate did not emerge in the public imagination until Huxley's death some thirty years later (Brooke, 2001).

Once again, there were numerous local factors that might have contributed to the legend of Huxley soundly defeating Wilberforce in the debate over Darwin's theory, not the least of these factors is the fact that there was indeed a struggle developing at the time between clergy and scientists. The struggle, however, was centered on the desire of the scientists, such as Huxley, to be autonomous from the established Church. Up until this time, much scientific work was done by the clergy. By the mid-nineteenth century, there was a growing interest in making the practice of science more of a profession in its own right. New standards of rigor and training for scientists, standards that clergy could not meet, were proposed in an attempt, in part, to separate science from religion. This movement toward autonomy of science was opposed by the clergy who had, up until that time, been very influential in science and who saw the study of nature as part of their religious calling. Related to this was a developing rivalry between scientists and the clergy as to who should speak on scientific matters to the rest of society. The clergy were a privileged group in British society up to the nineteenth century. By mid-century, however, the privileges of the clergy were beginning to wane, thanks in no small part to the scientists who were more than a little jealous of the place the clergy held in the culture of the day (Brooke, 2001). These factors of time and location influenced the development of much of the legend surrounding the Wilberforce–Huxley debate of 1860, but legend has become truth for many people as they look at this event and see it as another clear example of religion trying, unsuccessfully, to keep scientific truth suppressed.

How did the Church and Christianity in general respond to Darwin's theory of evolution? Published in 1859, the theory made a case for creation by lawful and natural processes (Darwin, 1859/2003). Natural selection, according to Darwin, is the driving force of all biological development, and of human origins as well. Some theologians and Christian scientists condemned Darwin, and his theory of evolution became for them a great source of antagonism between science and religion. Geologist William Dawson and zoologist Louis Agassiz were well-known anti-Darwinists of the nineteenth century. Princeton Seminary theologian Charles Hodge argued that Darwinism was incompatible with creation guided by God. The very authority of the Bible was at stake for Hodge, and one had to choose between God's design of creation and Darwin's evolutionary theory.

Other theologians and Christian scientists, though, saw no or minimal problem with the evolutionary theory proposed by Darwin. James McCosh, president of Princeton University, was an evangelical minister who believed that evolutionary theory was not incompatible with Christian theology or with the idea of supernatural design. Another supporter of Darwin's theory was Henry Ward Beecher, one of the greatest preachers of the nineteenth century. For Beecher, evolutionary theory was consistent with the idea of social progress and improvement in the human condition, positions that Beecher championed. Harvard University botanist Asa Gray was an early proponent of Darwin's evolutionary theory in the United States. A devout and pious Christian, Gray adopted Darwin's ideas regarding the changeability of species. What we might now call a Christian evolutionist, Gray believed that natural selection was not inconsistent with theology. Indeed, for Gray, science and religion make a consistent whole; the very process of evolution was the object of God's design. In this respect, Gray was in agreement with another Princeton theologian, B.B. Warfield. While rejecting a purely reductionistic and naturalistic evolutionary theory, Warfield nevertheless believed that evolutionary theories that maintained design (this would not include Darwin's theory) helped explain the physical world.

As these examples show, the Christian response to Darwin was not universal condemnation. There was a range of reactions to Darwin's theory, making the simplistic notion of conflict and warfare untenable. For many, a clear break between religion and science was the only way (for example, Thomas Huxley); for others, however, Darwin's theory offered an opportunity to forge a new understanding of nature and how God works within the created order.

A final example of how many people see religion and science relating is the trial of John Scopes in 1925, the events of which were made famous by the play, and later the movie, *Inherit the Wind*. In the movie, Bertram Cates (the John Scopes character) is a young biology teacher at a small-town high school. Led by the narrow-minded local minister, the sheriff arrests Cates in his classroom and puts him in jail for teaching evolution to his impressionable students. Tried for violating a state law forbidding such teaching, the Scopes character is defended by a smart, polite, reasonable, understanding and kind attorney played by Spencer Tracy. The prosecuting team is led by the dislikeable, loud, arrogant and intolerant attorney played by Fredric March. The townspeople are made to look like ignorant rubes as the movie unfolds, with the hymn 'Give Me That Old Time Religion, It's Good Enough For Me' playing in the background. Again, religion pays a heavy price when it goes up against science. The young teacher is indeed found guilty by the jury, but only after the Tracy character makes the prosecuting attorney look hopelessly foolish and ill-informed.

The reality of the events surrounding the Scopes trial is quite different, as detailed in the Edward Larson book *Summer for the Gods*, winner of the 1998 Pulitzer Prize in History (Larson, 1997). As detailed by Larson, the arrest and trial of Scopes was a well-planned publicity stunt by some of the prominent citizens of Dayton (including the local school board president and school superintendent). Seen as a way of getting much-needed attention for the town, these officials sought out Scopes and asked him if he would be willing to challenge the state's law on the teaching of evolution. (Scopes taught general science, not biology, and it is not clear how much Scopes knew about evolutionary theory or whether he even mentioned it in any of his classes.) Scopes agreed, and was defended by the American Civil Liberties Union and the most famous trial lawyer of the time, Clarence Darrow. A well-known defender of labor organizers and political radicals, Darrow was opposed to any religious influence in public life. For Darrow, there was no place for religion in the public square, in part because he believed it divided people. He was especially opposed to biblical literalism, which he saw as irrational and dangerous. Defending Scopes (and evolutionary theory) offered Darrow the chance to debunk the biblical notions of creation, design and purpose in nature. His intent was not so much to get Scopes declared not guilty of violating the state law, but to challenge the law itself.

The prosecution of Scopes was led by William Jennings Bryan, three-time Democratic nominee for President of the United States. While a political progressive, Bryan was conservative in his religion, and he saw Darwinism as potential support for excessive militarism, imperialism and *laissez-faire* capitalism, three ideas he found unacceptable and fought throughout his political career. In addition, Bryan saw the kind of legislation passed in Tennessee as a way to solve social problems exacerbated by evolutionary theory (for example, immorality). With Bryan and Darrow as the attorneys, the trial of John Scopes became the most celebrated event of the early twentieth century, receiving tremendous national interest. Every national and regional paper followed the trail; WGN radio out of Chicago covered it live.

The climax of the trial came with Bryan taking the stand and defending the anti-evolution statute. Bryan also wanted to protect revealed religion and biblical literalism against the attacks of Darrow, who for his part wanted to show the ignorance of Bryan and of those who supported both biblical literalism and the state law. Darrow's cross-examination of Bryan ended in a shouting match, and the judge suspended the proceedings. The jury found Scopes guilty, he was fined $100 by the judge, and Bryan died a few days later. (Bryan College was founded in Dayton in his honor. Classes at the college began in 1930.) The verdict, however, was overturned by the Tennessee Supreme Court, and Scopes went off to the University of Kentucky and then to the University of Chicago to study geology. (While Scopes's conviction was overturned, the anti-evolutionist position won the day, in that one of the long-term results of the trial was an exclusion of any discussion of evolutionary theory in biology textbooks in the United States for many years.)

The Scopes trial is used to show how religion is eventually superseded by scientific rationality. As with the other two examples, however, there is as much myth and legend to these stories as there is fact. This brief history of relations between science and religion is not meant to be inclusive. There are many books on this topic that can be read for a thorough and detailed historical account of how science and religion have been studied and understood in the past.[1] The purpose of this quick history is to highlight how our perspective of science and religion might be affected by erroneous information. In each of the cases mentioned above, there is as much myth as fact (perhaps more). Each of these examples represents one way of approaching the relationship between science and religion. This perspective is one of conflict, and is the first of the four models developed by Ian Barbour to try to understand and study how science and religion relate. In the next section of this chapter, Barbour's typologies will be explained and proposed as useful models that one can employ in thinking about science and religion.

Barbour's Typologies

Ian Barbour (b. 1923) seemed to have an interest in both science and religion early in his career. With an undergraduate degree in physics, Barbour went on to obtain a PhD in high-energy physics from the University of Chicago. After a few years of teaching physics in college, Barbour enrolled in the Yale Divinity School and also took classes at Union Seminary in New York City. In 1955, Barbour went to Carleton College in Minnesota and taught courses in both the departments of physics and religion. He has written several books on the theological implications of scientific theories (for example, the Big Bang and quantum physics), but his 1966 book *Issues in Science and Religion* is credited by many with creating the contemporary field of science and religion study. In 1990, Barbour's Gifford Lectures were published in *Religion in an Age of Science*, and this book was later revised as *Religion and Science: Historical and Contemporary Issues* in 1997. It is in these two books that

1 There are several excellent introductory books to science and religion which emphasize the complexity of the issues, including Brooke (1991), Ferngren (2002) and Lindberg and Numbers (1986, 2003).

Barbour lays out his four models or typologies of how science and religion might be seen to 'go together'.

The first of Barbour's typologies is Conflict. This model sees a basic incompatibility and discord between science and religion, and is indicative of the approach described in the examples above (for example, the received view of the Galileo Affair). Barbour sees two basic forms of the Conflict model, one represented by scientific materialism, and one by biblical literalists. Francis Crick, Daniel Dennett and Richard Dawkins are individuals who hold a scientific materialist view according to which science is the only way to acquire knowledge because only material things exist. There is only one reality, a material reality, and only methods designed to study that material reality (that is, science) are legitimate. Religion, which is interested in a nonexistent immaterial reality, can contribute nothing to the pursuit of truth and knowledge, so can be completely ignored.

Biblical literalists, according to Barbour, also see a basic conflict between religion and science. One individual representing this view is Ken Ham, a founder of the organization Answers in Genesis, which uses a literal interpretation of Genesis to show how not only evolutionary theory, but other scientific theories as well are in error. Another person who held this view was Henry Morris (1919–2006), a former director of the Institute for Creation Research and one of the leading proponents of the position known as creationism. For Ham (and Morris before his death), the Bible is understood as a literal description of how God created the heavens and the earth, and is the ultimate authority for all truth, including scientific truth (Giberson and Yerxa, 2002, pp. 67–83). Scientific ideas, such as the Big Bang, evolution, or an old earth, are in contradiction to this literal reading, and therefore not accepted. Both the scientific materialists and the biblical literalists agree that there is little hope for any reconciliation between science and religion. Richard Dawkins and Ken Ham would agree that Darwinism leads to atheism. For Dawkins, that move to atheism is intellectually satisfying and embraced; for Ham and other biblical literalists, it is a sign of how science can threaten fundamental religious (and ultimately moral) beliefs and practices.

The second of Barbour's typologies is Independence. In this model, both science and religion are separate domains, each with its own methods and language. It is sometimes said that science studies the natural world using empirical methods based upon experience, and answers questions about how creation works and how the universe came into existence. Religion, on the other hand, is interested in questions such as why there is a universe, is there a purpose to creation, and who is the creator – questions unanswerable using the methods of science. There is within the Christian tradition a long history of speaking about the Two Books of God, the Book of Special Revelation (the Bible) and the Book of General Revelation (nature). Each of these sources of data is from God, and therefore true (God is the source of all truth), and one book is not more true than the other (God's truth does not vary in degree), so there can be no conflict between what the Special Revelation says and what the General Revelation tells us. Both of these books, however, must be interpreted. Scientists interpret the book of nature using the language of science, and theologians (or biblical scholars) interpret the Bible using the language of religion. There could be a conflict between what science tells us about an issue (for example, the creation of the universe) and what theologians tell us, because both scientists and theologians are human and are subject to making erroneous observations and statements. Conflict cannot, however, exist between the two sources of data, the Special and the General Revelation.

Some within this position argue that while a scientific account of creation and a religious account are independent, they are nevertheless compatible and complementary. Because the two books provide answers to different kinds of questions (for example, how versus who and why), one needs to consider both the religious and the scientific perspective in order to have a complete picture of what God has created, why he has created, and how he has created. This multiple perspective is necessary to avoid what some have called 'nothing buttery', the reductionistic position typical of scientific materialism, that once one has understood the how of creation (the scientific story), one has learned all there is to know. The multiple-perspectives position also recognizes the limitations of both science and theology. Theology is limited to answering questions about what some have termed primary or ultimate causes (for example, God). Science, on the other hand, is limited to attempting to answer empirical questions, questions about naturalistic mechanisms or immediate (secondary) causes (for example, the Big Bang). Both types of questions need to be answered, and different perspectives are required to answer them. Although science and religion represent independent realms, methods and explanations, they relate in that they are complimentary approaches to studying what God has made.

The third typology of Barbour's goes beyond the notion of independent domains, and allows for and encourages greater Dialogue between science and religion. This dialogue can take place because there are times when science addresses questions, called boundary or limit questions by Barbour, to which religion also provides some answers. An example of such a limit question centers on the problem of why there is order and intelligibility in the universe. Why is the universe so orderly and lawful? Why are humans able to discern so much of how the universe works? Christian theology provides a possible explanation for these qualities in its formulation of the doctrine of creation which identifies who the creator is and why he created anything at all. Also part of this doctrine is the important idea that humans, being made in God's image, can share in a part of divine intelligibility. We can learn something about how the universe works and think God's thoughts after him because we have the *imago Dei*. Without this important contribution from the Judeo-Christian tradition, explaining order and intelligibility is left to random chance and statistical probability. Those explanations might be correct, but they do not have any *a priori* preference over the equally non-empirical and non-scientific account provided via the doctrine of creation.

Another way science and religion can enter into dialogue comes from the recognition that science and religion are not as different methodologically as was once thought to be the case and as is implied in the Independence typology. This is not to suggest that the methods of religion and science are the same; they certainly are not. It is to suggest, however, that the old approach that understood science as completely objective, impersonal and sterile, and whose theories are totally determined by empirically collected data, is no longer held. From this newer perspective, known as *postpositivism*, scientific theories are seen as underdetermined by data, and the scientific process is unavoidably more subjective and personal than once thought (see Chapter 4). There is therefore greater overlap between religion and, for example, psychological science than earlier theologians or scientists believed (Jones, 1994), making a dialogue between the two mutually beneficial.

The final typology of Barbour's is Integration, where science and religion go beyond dialogue to the point of influencing and, perhaps, modifying each other. One example of integration is natural theology, which has a long history traceable at least to the work of Thomas Aquinas. The basic claim of natural theology is that 'the existence of God can be inferred from the evidences of design in nature, of which science has made us more aware' (Barbour, 1997, p. 98). Scientists tell us that there are hundreds of cosmological constants (for example, the rotation speed of the earth, distance of the earth from the sun, the gravitational force) that are seemingly 'fine-tuned' to enable life on earth (Barrow, 2003). Changing any one of these independent constants by the smallest of percentage points would make life on earth impossible. Other scientists have observed a trend toward increased complexity in life, an inevitable, convergent and emergent pattern of life evolving into intelligent life (Morris, 2003). This kind of evidence can be taken, although not necessarily so, to suggest a design and purpose to existence. The existence of God is a hypothesis with a certain probability, and this probability increases or decreases with obtained evidence from nature. Natural theology suggests that the evidence of nature points more and more strongly to support for the God hypothesis.

A second example of Integration is known as theology of nature, which begins with theology and looks to science to see whether any theological doctrines might be modified in light of scientific findings. For example, in what ways might the traditional philosophical and theological concept of the soul be reformed in response to contemporary findings coming from psychology and neuroscience which emphasize the emergent properties of personhood and a holistic self?[2] (This question will be addressed in Chapter 7.) Other issues where a theology of nature might be applicable are on the question of human freedom and the classical ideas of God's omnipotence and omniscience. Theology is not, or should not be, a static and never-changing discipline. In the tradition of the reformers, contemporary theology should seek to engage science (and philosophy) in an attempt to speak to contemporary culture, all the while remaining true to biblical intuitions about God's relation to the world (Shults, 2005, pp. 9–12, 201).

Other Approaches

Evolution, meaning change in species, is a phenomenon that was well known before Darwin. What Darwin did in 1859 was provide a plausible explanation for the fact of evolution that involved random genetic variation and natural selection. As discussed above, some clergy embraced Darwin's ideas and saw them as compatible with

2 The important question of how the traditional concept of the soul can be reformed in response to contemporary findings in psychology and neuroscience is considered in Green (2004a), Habgood (1998), Jeeves (2004a) and Shults (2003).

Christian theology, while others rejected these naturalistic processes as atheistic and contrary to established Christian beliefs regarding creation. There is still disagreement today about how or whether evolutionary theories (Darwin's theory is only one of many attempts to explain the processes of evolution) can be brought into some kind of dialogue or even integration with theology. While some theologians and clergy, particularly in the United States, see all evolutionary theories (but perhaps especially Darwin's) as antithetical to Judeo-Christian tradition and belief, others seek to go beyond merely seeing evolution as compatible with Christian theology, and see the possibility of a kind of evolutionary theology where Darwin's theory actually elucidates Christian theology's idea of God. An example of such an approach is provided by John Haught, Professor of Theology at Georgetown University. In *God After Darwin*, Haught proposes that Darwin's two dangerous ideas – that all living beings share a common ancestry, and that the processes of evolution are completely naturalistic and undirected by any intelligent agency – represent not only a challenge, but also a great gift to theology. It is a gift because Darwin's theory enables theology to reclaim certain features of the Christian faith that were neglected and forgotten with all of the talk of design and order in nature. Yes, there is order within creation, but there is also novelty, and this feature of nature suggests that the cosmos is an unfinished process, much like evolution. According to Haught, evolutionary theory (even a neo-Darwinian evolutionary account) gives us insights into the nature of God's relationship to his creation. Influenced by the work of Teilhard de Chardin and emphasizing an eschatological perspective of creation, Haught suggests that this evolutionary informed theology supports the biblical notion of a new heaven and a new earth with God drawing all of creation to himself from 'up ahead'. Instead of a rigid plan for creation, evolutionary theory enables God's 'vision' for the universe which promises a new being and a new creation. Rather than eliminating meaning and purpose from life, Darwin's theory illuminates the biblical image of God, and viewing the evolutionary data in the light of this biblical image makes more sense than seeing the same data through the lens of scientific materialism (Haught, 2000, p. 47).

Another recent example of putting science and religion together is the work of Alister McGrath, a doctorally trained biophysicist and Professor of Historical Theology at Oxford University. McGrath believes that 'the working methods and assumptions of the natural sciences can stimulate and inform the working methods and assumptions of a responsible Christian theology' (McGrath, 2004b, p. 22). A positive relationship between Christian theology and the natural sciences is demanded by the Christian doctrine of the creation, according to McGrath, because the God of Christian theology is the same God who created the natural world that natural scientists study. Natural science, therefore, is an *ancilla theologiae* or handmaiden to theology, helping theology understand the God of creation. As summarized in *The Science of God* (McGrath, 2004b) and extensively explored and developed in the three volumes of *A Scientific Theology* (McGrath, 2001, 2002, 2003), scientific theology is a 'style of theology which arises out of an engagement with the natural sciences' rather than with some specific scientific theory which can change with time (McGrath, 2004b, p. 23). Based on traditional Christian orthodoxy (for example, the incarnation and the doctrine of creation) and a realist perspective of God (that is, God is real, and is not a construction or projection of the human mind), scientific theology is an attempt to integrate science and religion at the deep level of method and assumptions. It represents a Christian theology enriched by the natural sciences coming from a scholar with unquestioned credentials in both natural science and theology.

The Current Scene

While the conflict and warfare view of the relationship between science and religion has been thoroughly discredited, it nevertheless remains part of the culture, at least in the United States. It is currently raising its ugly head in the ongoing 'debate' between evolution and the most recent version of 'creationism' known as intelligent design (ID) (see Dembski and Ruse, 2004; Pennock, 2001). It has been convincingly argued that this controversy is a North American phenomenon, and that in other parts of the world (for example, Europe), 'creationism' as it is typically understood in the United States does not exist and ID is unheard of (Staune, 2005). (Ron Numbers (2006 p. 399), however, has recently argued that creationism is now a global phenomenon that has adherents not only in Protestantism, but also in Eastern Orthodoxy, Islam and Hinduism.). While the controversy in Europe might be over the processes of evolution (Darwinian or non-Darwinian), the debates in the United States are at a more fundamental (and heated) level, most recently played out in Dover, Pennsylvania, where the local School Board voted in 2004 to require ninth-grade biology students to be made aware of problems with Darwin's theory of evolution and to also be taught alternative theories of origins such as ID. Some parents of the affected students sued the school board, arguing that the teaching of intelligent design violated the Establishment Clause of the United States Constitution. The case went to federal court (*Kitzmiller* v. *Dover*), where the judge ruled, in December of 2005, that the School Board policy did violate the Establishment Clause, and that based on the evidence presented in court, ID could not be taught in the biology classroom as an alternative scientific theory to evolution. The judge in the case determined that intelligent design was tied to creationism, and therefore to religion.

Proponents of ID had maintained that, once the theory was considered in court, the evidence would show that it was, indeed, a science. Some of the leading figures in the ID movement, for example Michael Behe, biologist at Leheigh University, testified in the case, as did recognized authorities on the other side of the issue. One of the scientists who testified in favor of the parents was Kenneth Miller, a biologist from Brown University, who is the coauthor of a widely used high school biology textbook as well as the author of *Finding Darwin's God*, a book seeking to reconcile Darwin's theory with belief in a creator God (Miller, 1999). The fact that the judge ruled against ID was considered a great victory and vindication to the anti-ID position, and an unjust decision by an activist judge by the losing side. The voters of Dover, Pennsylvania, chose a new School Board at the next election, replacing all members who had previously voted to include the teaching of ID in the science curriculum. The entire incident illustrates the volatile nature of the issue, at least in the United States, and shows how much of the general public, as well as many scientists, still persist in seeing science and religion in conflict despite the work of historians like Brooke and scientists like Miller who argue that conflict is neither historically accurate nor scientifically necessary.

Thus far, we have examined some basic principles in neuroscience, psychology and religion, and seen how the philosophy of science has changed from a very objective and impersonal positivistic approach to a more subjective and personal postpositivistic view. In the remaining chapters, we will consider particular topics where neuroscience, psychology and religion can 'come together' into a kind of dialogue, or even a type of integration. As we examine these areas of interaction, we will approach them from the assumption that reality is multileveled or stratified (Looy, Reimer and Seybold, 2005). As a result, we must use multiple methods and approaches to understand the complexities of human experience. While reality is multileveled, it is also a whole; by recognizing reality as a multileveled whole, we hope to avoid making the mistake of 'nothing buttery', as too often occurs when studying a subject scientifically.

Trying to bring science and religion together into a dialogue, or even integration, is not easy. It is and should be difficult, because for Christians and people of other faith traditions, religious beliefs are important. These beliefs hopefully guide our lives, influence the decisions we make, and affect the way we relate to others. We are Christians (or we identify with another religious tradition), in part, because Christianity works for us. In addition, however, we believe that the teachings of Jesus Christ are true. Our faith is not something we can, or should, ignore; it is an important part of our lives. Science is also important for many Christians, and as the Habgood quote at the beginning of this chapter suggests, it is possible to be both an honest Christian and an honest scientist. It is in this spirit that we continue our exploration of neuroscience, psychology and religion.

Chapter 6

Brain and Religion

Along with about five hundred others and accompanied by a piano and organ, I was standing and singing 'How Great Thou Art' in the morning worship service of my home church. As I did so, I felt something special happen. I felt what many would describe as a religious experience; I sensed God's presence in a way that I did not feel a few minutes earlier. While no one watching me would have noticed any change in what I was experiencing, it was nevertheless real to me. Others in the congregation lifted their hands during the song, the expressions on their faces suggesting pleasure, or even ecstasy. Had I been in another church, I might have seen worshipers dancing, heard them shouting or speaking in tongues, or perhaps falling to the ground in a kind of trance-like state. A friend of mine tells of his conversion experience, during which he felt real physical pain throughout his body, spoke to Jesus in as real a way as he would speak to his wife, and when he asked Jesus if he could see his face, saw the faces of members of his wife's church who had been praying for him for many years.

What accounts for these kinds of occurrences? Are religious experiences different from other experiences we might have at sporting events, parties or holiday celebrations? Are they religious only because they take place in a particular setting (for example, at church during worship), or are these kinds of experiences religious because they are different in some essential and fundamental way? How does God 'make his presence known' to believers – through some unique path only he uses, or by the same pathways through which we become aware of the world around us?

These questions are fundamental in any attempt to look at religion, psychology and the neurosciences. Everything we do, think, feel, desire, sense and so on is accomplished using the brain, so to answer these questions, we need to understand something of how this brain of ours works. What follows is a simplified version of the workings of the nervous system, but it is hopefully enough to allow us to discuss and understand how the brain is the organ for all of our experiences, physical, mental, and perhaps even spiritual.

The Nervous System

The building block of the nervous system is the nerve cell or neuron. In some ways, neurons are like other cells of the body. For example, neurons have a nucleus which contains the genetic material of the cell. Neurons also have structures that enable the cell to produce energy, get rid of waste, and move materials from one part of the neuron to another. Unlike other bodily cells, however, neurons are different in that they can generate an electrical message. It is this property that makes nerve cells unique and so important in our ability to experience the world around us. It is by way of these electrical messages that we are able to know our external world, our own physical condition, and even our own thoughts and wishes.

As described more fully in Chapter 1, neurons have four main parts. First is the *cell body* (or soma). This component of the neuron contains the nucleus and many of the structures referred to above that are common to all cells of the body. The second feature of the neuron is the *axon*, which leaves the cell body and connects the neuron to other nerve cells. Near its end, the axon begins to divide, and eventually terminates in what are called *terminal buttons*. Finally, *dendrites* are the branch-like features seen in Figure 1.1.

As mentioned above, neurons are different from other cells of the body in that they generate electrical impulses (or neural impulses), and these electrical messages are produced by the movement of ions into and out of the neuron. The movement of ions into or out of the neuron occurs through openings or 'channels' in the neuron's membrane, a structure that defines the boundary of the cell. The most important of these ions (charged molecules) are sodium (Na^+), potassium (K^+), and chloride (Cl^-). As indicated, some of these ions are positively charged and some negatively charged, and whether they are positively or negatively charged is important in influencing the generation of the neural impulse. If enough positively charged ions (most importantly Na^+) enter a neuron, it becomes excited and is likely to generate this electrical impulse. If enough negatively charged ions enter a neuron, it is inhibited and is less likely to generate the impulse. So whether or not an electrical message is produced depends primarily upon the movement of these ions in and out of the neuron.

While neurons normally do not make physical contact with other neurons, they do communicate with each other at the synapse, a 'functional' connection between one nerve cell and another. Typically, the synapse (see Figure 1.2) is between the terminal button of the neuron sending the message and the dendrite of the neuron receiving the message. A small gap, approximately 20 nm (billionth of a meter) wide, exists between the terminal button and the dendrite. When the electrical message arrives at the synapse, it causes the release of a chemical (called a neurotransmitter) from the terminal button. This neurotransmitter travels across the synaptic cleft and stimulates the dendrite of the receiving neuron. If this stimulation increases the flow of positively charges ions into the receiving neuron, then that nerve cell is more likely to generate its own electrical message, which is sent down its axon to the next nerve cell. In this way, information is sent from one part of the nervous system to another. (See Chapter 1 for a more complete description of the process of communication within the nervous system.)

How Do We Experience the World?

> What is real? How do you define real? If you're talking about what you can feel, what you can smell, what you can taste and see, then real is simply electrical signals interpreted by your brain. This is the world that you know. (Morpheus's response to Neo about reality in the 1999 movie *The Matrix*)

The brain is involved in all of our behavior and experience. All that we do, think, feel or believe involves the brain in some way. In the nineteenth century, psychologists and other scientists began to understand how we encounter the world through our senses, particularly the senses of vision and audition. Along with advances made during that century in optics and acoustics, these psychologists clarified how light and sound energy are changed, or transduced, into electrical impulses that carry the visual and auditory information through the brain. In the twentieth century, advances were made in detailing how other sensory information (for example, touch, taste and smell) was also processed.

In order to detect sensory information in the environment, it is necessary to have receptors sensitive to a particular kind of energy (light, sound, chemical and so on) and that the energy be of sufficient intensity to stimulate the receptors into generating electrical impulses (the process of sensation). Once that electrical message is produced, it is carried along the neurons of the nervous system until it reaches specific regions of the brain where the electrical impulses begin to be 'interpreted' (the process of perception). We are sensitive to a variety of kinds of energy in our environment; however, all energy is changed into electrical impulses within the nervous system. The term 'representation' is used to describe how objects in our environment are experienced in the brain; they are represented in the form of patterns of these neural impulses.

Emotion and thinking are also products, in part, of electrical impulses reaching specific brain areas or being generated within those areas. Movement, too, is produced by electrical impulses generated in specific brain regions and sent to the muscles of our body. Even our own body is represented in the brain. Portions of the brain surface (or cortex) contain areas that 'represent' various parts of the human body. If electrical impulses originate from the big toe and reach the portion of the cortex devoted to the big toe, we feel a sensation in that part of our body. The phantom limb phenomenon occurs in many individuals who have experienced the amputation of a limb, for example a foot. Despite the amputation, these individuals experience sensation in the foot because electrical impulses are still arriving at the 'foot' area of the brain.

This relationship between external stimulus and the generated electrical impulses that make up inner perception has led some philosophers and scientists to question whether we can be sure that what we perceive is an accurate copy or representation of what is present in the external environment. Perceptual illusions, such as the moon illusion, where the moon appears larger on the horizon than it does at its peak position in the sky, illustrate how our perceptions can be wrong. However, even with the recognition that what we perceive and what we know are influenced by context and culture, there is general agreement among neuroscientists that these patterns of neural impulses are an accurate representation of the real world.

Cognition and Emotion

While emotion has been a topic of study in psychology for several decades, neuroscience has only recently begun to explore it. Using the latest brain imaging procedures, neuroscientists can take a picture of the brain while a person is experiencing a particular kind of emotion (for example, anger, happiness). What the neuroscientists are finding suggests that emotion plays a larger part in our thoughts and decisions than once believed. The seventeenth-century philosopher René Descartes separated mind (thought) from the body. Contemporary research on emotion, however, suggests that emotion is closely tied to our mental abilities, and even to our identity as individual persons.

One area of study looks at the role emotion plays in making decisions. A view known as the rationalist perspective suggests that we use logic and reason in making decisions, and that emotion plays no role at all. Haidt (2001) showed, however, that much of the reasoning connected to our decision making comes after our emotions point us toward a particular choice. In other words, emotional input to the decision comes before rational input. We use reason, it seems, to justify the decisions we make using our emotions.

Other studies on emotion suggest that even when we experience the so-called social emotions (for example, empathy) there are clear brain structures involved. Farrow and colleagues (2001) used a brain imaging procedure called functional MRI, and found that specific patterns of brain activity occurred when subjects made decisions to forgive or to empathize. Brain areas in the prefrontal cortex (PFC) and temporal lobe are also involved in social behaviors and moral emotions such as guilt and shame (Moll et al., 2002).

The PFC has many subdivisions, two of which, the orbitofrontal and dorsolateral sections, are clearly involved in the processing of emotions. It is also established that the left and right hemispheres, while working together, often process information in different ways. Some evidence suggests that positive emotions like happiness and joy involve the PFC in the left hemisphere, while the right PFC is involved in the processing of negative emotions such as sadness (Davidson and Irwin, 1999). The experience of emotion in individuals with damage to the PFC can therefore be affected. For example, a person with damage to the left PFC (positive emotions) might have difficulty recovering from negative events in his or her life because the brain area that processes positive emotions is not able to compensate for the overwhelming negative emotions produced by the right PFC in response to the person's life situation. The person experiences the negative emotion unchecked by the left PFC which would normally produce a balancing positive emotion in the individual.

The anticipation of future positive and negative emotional consequences also involves the PFC, and it is this area of the brain that was severely damaged in the well-known case of Phineas Gage. In September of 1848, near Cavendish, Vermont, Gage, who was a foreman for the railroad, was working clearing rock for a new railroad line. The process involved drilling a hole in the rock, pouring gunpowder into the hole, putting a fuse in the powder, and then covering the powder and fuse with sand. The last step before lighting the fuse was to tamp the sand into the hole with a 3–4-foot iron rod. On this particular day, Gage was perhaps distracted, and somehow neglected to put sand into the hole before he used the tamping rod. Sparks from the rod striking the rock ignited the gunpowder driving the rod through Gage's cheekbone, into his orbitofrontal cortex, and out his skull. Surprisingly, Gage never lost consciousness. He was taken to a doctor, who bandaged his wounds and, essentially, waited for Gage to die. While Gage's body survived the accident, he did nevertheless experience major personality changes, emotional instability (Davidson, Jackson and Kalin, 2000) and an inability to predict future emotional responses in himself or others. All of these changes disrupted his ability to plan effectively, interact in social environments, and show responsibility for himself or others. His friends remarked that after the accident, Gage was no longer himself. He became profane, impulsive and angry, characteristics that did not describe Gage before the accident. Early damage to the PFC (for example, during childhood) can also result in behavior symptomatic of psychopathology, including poor social interactions, decreased knowledge of how to act in social situations, diminished sense of guilt relative to behavior, and impaired sensitivity to rewards and punishments (Anderson et al., 1999).

Another brain structure involved in emotional processing is the amygdala, located in the temporal lobe. Joseph LeDoux of New York University has shown that the amygdala is vital in processing the emotion of fear (LeDoux, 1996). In particular, the amygdala helps in learning about new threats, evaluating a situation as threatening, and in the expression of fear (Amaral, 2002; Davidson, 2002).

Why is the study of emotion important to a discussion about religion and the brain? The University of Cambridge psychologist Fraser Watts, in writing about the centrality of emotion in religion, notes that both theologians and psychologists find a fundamental role for emotion in religion (Watts, 1997). One theologian from the nineteenth century (Schleiermacher) believed that emotion was the essence and source of religion, and the best way to determine the religiosity of an individual was to examine his or her emotional expression. Indeed, a study in 2002 found that cancer patients defined their religious faith using primarily positive rather than negative emotion words, suggesting that religious faith can be understood using emotion terminology (Ramírez-Johnson et al., 2002). Schleiermacher also believed that religious emotion was fundamentally different and distinct from other emotional experiences.

Writing at the beginning of the twentieth century, the influential philosopher and psychologist William James also emphasized the importance of emotion in religious experience. To James, however, emotions or feelings are a consequence of bodily states, and religious emotions are religious in nature because of the context in which the emotions occur. In other words, religious emotions are not different from other emotions; they are religious because of their religious references. James's position on emotion is supported by the findings of modern cognitive psychology and cognitive neuroscience, which suggest that the body is centrally involved in the creation of emotion. In fact, emotion is considered by some to be the body's chemical or hormonal response to a situation. Emotion is also thought to be important in thought, providing an appropriate context for emotion. Physiological responses are important in emotion and in religion (see below). Cognition also plays a role in both religious and emotional expression (Watts, 1997).

Ilkka Pyysiäinen is a comparative theologian at the Universities of Turku and Helsinki in Finland. He sees religion as a way of dealing with ideas that are inevitable but inappropriate explanations for events. Once formed, these ideas must be made coherent and organized, which is the function of religion. Dealing with these ideas, however, can produce emotions some of which can be extremely intense (for example, mystical experiences). So, like James, Pyysiäinen sees emotion as the basis of religious experience, and argues that it is correlated with a person's thoughts and cognitions (Pyysiäinen, 2001).

Neurotheology

As suggested above, scientists are clarifying the role the brain plays in emotion, and are shedding light on the connection between emotion and thought. Scientists are also studying the importance of thoughts and feelings in religious experience. In the 1990s, a new way of investigating religious experience emerged, called neurotheology. Eugene d'Aquili and Andrew Newberg (1999, p. 18), leading researchers in this area, define neurotheology as how the mind/brain functions in terms of one's relationship to God or ultimate reality. The role of the brain in religious experience and in our relating to God is an important topic, and is one that has captured the attention of scientists, theologians and laypeople alike. The cover story of the 7 May 2001 *Newsweek* magazine was entitled 'God and the Brain', and a variety of books on the topic can be found in any large bookstore. Some people might fear that neurotheology is an attempt to 'prove' the existence (or nonexistence) of God, or to find where God is 'located' in the brain. These fears are fueled by statements made by some scientists suggesting that God is 'nothing more' than some electrical blip in the brain. The existence of God, of course, must be taken, ultimately, on faith; it is not a question that can be answered by science. The scientific study of religious phenomena, however, can tell us something about what is occurring physiologically when we have a religious or spiritual experience.

One of the first scientists to study the brain's involvement in religious experience was Michael Persinger, who in the early 1980s published articles dealing with religious experiences and brain activity, and by the end of that decade published a book on the neuropsychology of God beliefs (Persinger, 1987). Persinger emphasized the role of a particular region of the brain (the temporal lobe) in normal religious as well as mystical experiences. One reason for looking to the temporal lobe as a source of these experiences, argues Persinger, is because it is electrically unstable, which can produce activity in the structure that does not necessarily correspond to real sensory input. An unstable temporal lobe allows for the possibility of confusion or a mixture of current experience and fantasy. The temporal lobe is also a well-known site of seizure activity (or epilepsy), which often accompanies hallucinations. According to Persinger, religious experience is caused by short-term electrical abnormalities within the temporal lobe. In more extreme cases of these seizures, behavioral signs might emerge, such as crying, facial distortions, speaking in tongues and amnesia.

We are able, says Persinger, to have an experience of God because the temporal lobe developed the way it did. Had the structures within the temporal lobe developed differently, the 'God experience would not have occurred' (Persinger, 1987, p. 14). Persinger believes that the experience of God, because it is merely a biological artifact of the brain, can be controlled by others, and he is concerned about the many people who have died or been killed waiting for, or as a result of, these seizures. Persinger goes on to say that various stimuli sometimes found in religious settings (for example, music, certain body movements like swaying and dancing, repetitive sounds, and odors) can trigger temporal lobe seizures. Despite such dramatic statements, Persinger does not provide much scientific evidence to support his fundamental hypothesis. While providing confirmation for the temporal lobe as a target for seizure activity, he does not supply evidence for statements more directly referring to his belief that religious experience is a mere artifact of such seizure activity. Nor does he offer support when he likens belief in God to a 'cognitive virus' and delusion (Persinger, 2002, pp. 279–81).

Rhawn Joseph also believes that limbic system structures (the amygdala, hippocampus and inferior temporal lobe) provide the foundation for spiritual and religious experience, and suggests that the apparent universality of religious belief is due to the commonality of the limbic system to all people. Similar brain structures and organization lead to universal religious and spiritual experience. These same brain structures are also involved in sexuality, rage and sadistic behavior, so it is understandable, Joseph argues, that the God of the Old Testament should be 'inordinately concerned with sexuality, is often enraged, and requires the experience of fear in which to reveal divine presence and power' (Joseph, 2001, p. 118). It is, suggests Joseph, because of activation of the limbic system that religious people are many times also hateful, belligerent and murderous.

Despite offering these rather reductionistic explanations, Joseph acknowledges that science cannot rule out the possibility that the brain structures and networks implicated in religious experience might have evolved because there is a spiritual world. So while the limbic system might metaphorically be considered the seat of the soul or some point of contact with God, this 'transmitter to God' could, Joseph speculates, increase the likelihood of survival because it helps the individual make contact with reality (in this case, a spiritual reality), as do other evolved structures and networks in the brain (Joseph, 2001, p. 132).

Another researcher who is looking at how the brain is involved in religious experience is Carol Albright, who cautions against overly reductionistic accounts of religious experience. Locating a 'God module' or 'transmitter to God' in limbic system structures ignores the fact, according to Albright, that the brain operates as a whole, not as unrelated and independent modules. While there is some localization of function in the human nervous system, the popular idea that the brain consists of several totally independent areas, or the commonly held view that the brain actually consists of two brains – a right brain and a left brain – is not an accurate view of this organ at all. In reality, the brain operates as a result of complex interconnections among these modules or areas. It would be more correct to say, therefore, that the entire brain is involved in religious or God experiences (Albright, 2000). Religious experience is multifaceted, so we should expect it to activate the brain in a variety of ways and in a variety of areas.

Despite operating holistically, Albright and her colleague James Ashbrook do recognize three basic levels or kinds of areas in the human nervous system: the reptilian brain, the mammalian brain, and the neocortex. Each of these major regions is, in Albright and Ashbrook's theory, associated with various beliefs and perceptions about God (Ashbrook and Albright, 1997). The reptilian brain is responsible for behaviors humans share with reptiles, such as protection of self and territory, reproduction, feeding and so on. These behaviors often lead humans into difficulty and trouble, so must, in some way, be 'civilized'. Religious practices and beliefs traditionally provide guidance to people regarding raising children, sexual behavior and violence, and are seen as attempts to bring this reptilian brain under control. In addition, the authors suggest that images and ideas of a watchful, persistent, unchanging God might reflect the activity of this reptilian part of the human brain.

The mammalian brain consists of the limbic system, which adds emotion to the functions provided by the reptilian brain, and emotion helps to identify safe or unsafe behaviors. The limbic system is also largely responsible for memory. With memory and emotion, we are able to develop, according to Ashbrook and Albright, a meaningful relationship with God.

Surrounding these two parts of the brain is the cerebral cortex, which provides much of what most people consider to be humanness, including language. It is also the area where much of the information processed at other brain regions converges so we can make decisions and judgments. Religious experience will involve each of these areas: mystical experience, love and kinship, the limbic system; rituals of various kinds, the reptilian brain; and discernment and a sense of calling from God, the cerebral cortex (for example, the frontal lobe).

Patrick McNamara, Professor of Psychiatry at Boston University School of Medicine, argues that religious practices are associated with activation of the frontal lobes, particularly the prefrontal cortex, which mediates what are known as executive cognitive functions, or ECFs (McNamara, 2001, p. 238). The frontal lobes are one of the last brain regions to mature, not fully developing until late adolescence. One of the ECFs important in religious practice, according to McNamara, is Theory of Mind, which is a postulated mechanism that enables one to attribute mental states to other persons or agents (for example, God). A person with a developed Theory of Mind would be able to predict the actions, beliefs and thoughts of others, and thus determine their intentions. The frontal lobes also participate directly in emotional processing, pro-social behavior, empathy and self-consciousness. These executive cognitive functions are also involved in the practice of religion. Theory of Mind enables one to develop a concept of God, implying to McNamara that damage to prefrontal cortex should impair one's understanding of God (a hypothesis that McNamara has as yet not tested empirically). Frontal lobe damage would also, according to this approach, produce impaired participation in the emotional aspects of religious experience, weakened self-control or self-discipline associated with religious beliefs and practices, and impoverished religious behaviors such as compassion and forgiveness. Being a mature and freely choosing human being requires intact and functioning frontal lobes. McNamara suggests that cultures promote those activities that serve as aids to help the frontal lobes develop and mature, and the near universality of religious practices (for example, prayer and meditation) acts as a means to accomplish this maturation (McNamara, 2002).

The frontal lobes, especially the prefrontal cortices, and the limbic system are also important in Antonio Damasio's somatic marker hypothesis. According to Damasio, bodily (or somatic) changes, such as hormonal and neural responses, provide feedback which marks a situation as either good, something to approach, or bad, something to avoid (Damasio, 1994, pp. 173–80). This automatic feedback, conditioned in part by culture, serves as a kind of 'gut reaction' which is used to develop a Theory of Mind and applied in making appropriate decisions, thus providing evolutionary advantage. The somatic marker hypothesis offers an alternative to McNamara's understanding of how religious practice seems nearly universal. Religious beliefs, attitudes and practices are part of this somatic marker system, and are evolutionarily adaptive because they provide a means of evaluating situations and making decisions.

Perhaps the most celebrated research on the neural basis of religious experience is that of Andrew Newberg, who, along with Eugene d'Aquili, brought this literature to a broader public awareness and led to cover stories in popular magazines like *Newsweek*. Newberg, and d'Aquili before his death, empirically investigated which brain areas are activated during religious experiences such as prayer in Franciscan nuns and Buddhists during meditation (Newberg and d'Aquili, 2001). Using a brain imaging technique called SPECT (Single Photon Emission Computed Tomography), which detects long-lasting radioactive tracers to measure the activity level of various brain structures and regions, an image of the brain can be taken several minutes after the tracer is injected into the brain. Newberg and d'Aquili injected the tracer at the peak of the religious experience, and were able to image the brain several minutes later. In this way, the imaging of the brain did not interfere with the religious experience itself.

Results from the Franciscan nuns and the Buddhist meditators were similar. An area in the parietal lobe near the top rear of the brain (the posterior superior parietal lobe) showed a decrease in activity during these peak religious experiences (as compared to activity level during a baseline period). The role of this part of the brain, according to Newberg, is to help us orient ourselves in space by generating a clear distinction between the self and the rest of the world. When this area is inhibited during prayer or meditation, the experience is reported as being close to God by the Franciscan nuns, and a sense of 'timelessness' or 'infinity' by the Buddhists. At the same time that areas of the parietal lobe decrease in activity, sites in the frontal lobe and limbic system increase in activity allowing, according to Newberg, for improved concentration, attention and focus during meditation and prayer. It is noted that these results are based on a limited sample of subjects. It is also important to remember that a neurobiological correlate to a subjective experience does not establish causality. Observing brain changes during a subjective spiritual experience does not mean that the brain activity is causing the experience. It might instead be the case that the spiritual experience is causing the brain changes, or that another unknown variable is producing both the changes in brain activity and the subjective experience. Despite these caveats, it is interesting that there seems to be some consistency in the brain areas involved in the practices of prayer and meditation, and the research by Newberg and his colleagues does represent a rare attempt by neuroscientists to empirically test hypotheses about the role of the brain in religious experience and goes beyond the speculation found in most of the literature.

Spirituality as an Innate Characteristic

What is the source of the seemingly universal tendency of humans to worship something? Is there, as some suggest, an innate spirituality that is a basic characteristic of the human species? Does the Christian doctrine of *imago Dei* imply that our destiny as human beings is to enter into fellowship with God, a destiny that is manifested here on earth as a drive to relate to something beyond ourselves (Shults, 1999, p. 224)?

Alister Hardy, a one-time zoologist at Oxford University, suggested that spirituality is a product of our biological nature. Hardy's hypothesis was that religious awareness, the divine flame as he called it, has survival value and evolved through a process of natural selection (Hardy, 1966, p. 27). More recently, another researcher from England, David Hay, suggests that children have a spirituality that cannot be explained by reference to environment or enculturation. In fact, Hay argues, it is enculturation into a secular society that suppresses the natural spirituality that is such a noticeable characteristic in children's lives (Hay and Nye, 1998, p. 18). Hay uses the term 'relational consciousness' to describe this biologically rooted spiritual awareness, which evolved, suggests Hay, because it promotes cooperation and a communal ethic, and allows, for the religious believer, a sense of relationship with God (Hay and Nye, 1998, pp. 141–7).

The recent report from the Commission on Children at Risk provides empirical evidence leading to the conclusion that children are hardwired to form connections with other people (parents, family, broader community) and are born with a built-in capacity to pursue questions closely linked with spirituality and religious belief (Commission on Children at Risk, 2003). Studies of twins at the University of Minnesota indicate that perhaps as much as 50 percent of religious interests, attitudes and values are influenced by genes (Waller et al., 1990), and Dean Hamer, a geneticist at the National Cancer Institute, maintains that human spirituality is 'hardwired into our genes', and is in fact a genetically encoded instinct (Hamer, 2004, p. 6). Hamer's 'God gene' turns out to be a variant of a gene that produces a protein involved in monoamine transmission in neurons. Monoamines are a family of compounds (such as norepinephrine, dopamine and serotonin) that are implicated in a variety of responses, including reward, reinforcement and emotion. Hamer (2004, pp. 72–3) found a statistically significant relationship between the presence of this variant, called VMAT2, and self-transcendence in a scale designed by Robert Cloninger to measure temperament and character. The self-transcendence measure has a number of sub-measures, including self-forgetfulness, transpersonal identification and mysticism, each of which is thought by Cloninger to be a component of spirituality. VMAT2 was most strongly associated with the self-forgetfulness subscale, and more weakly associated with the other two. (While Hamer emphasizes that genes do not act alone, that they have their effect through interacting with other genes as well as the environment, he nevertheless leaves the unfortunate impression that spirituality is ultimately reducible to the more basic levels of science, biology and chemistry.)

All of this evidence begs the question of why we seemingly have this innate spirituality. The renowned psychotherapist Sigmund Freud claimed that religious belief was an illusion, a kind of neurosis that should be treated like one would treat any psychological disorder. If Freud was right, why do humans seem to be biologically prepared to seek ultimate reality beyond ourselves and beyond the material world of which we are a part?

Evolutionary theory can be interpreted to suggest that the brain evolved these characteristics because, as apparently the only creatures aware of our own mortality, religious and spiritual beliefs serve to make our deaths more bearable. Religious experience, therefore, is a kind of 'built-in pacifier', to quote Michael Persinger in a *Time* magazine article (Chu et al., 2004, p. 68). However, one might also argue that if God exists and has created humans for the purpose of enjoying a relationship with him, a position consistent with traditional Christian theology, there should be some physical mechanism to allow for the development of that relationship. It should not be surprising, therefore, that the brain and the body in general have these kinds of physical structures or processes built-in to our biological nature.

Is God in the Brain?

What are we to make of the above research suggesting that certain brain areas (for example, the frontal lobe) are 'turned on' or 'light up' when a person has a religious experience such as praying? Some of the researchers involved go beyond the data and suggest that God can be found in these brain areas (the so-called 'God Spot'). To suggest, however, that God is located in the brain is no more accurate or acceptable than to say that the enjoyment of basketball is located in a 'Basketball Spot', or the experience of being moved by a play, painting or piece of music is located in a 'Fine Arts Spot'. Certainly, parts of the brain will 'light up' when a person enjoys watching a theater performance, but is that all there is to it? Yes, say some researchers like Persinger. Experiencing God *is* the stimulation of or activity in temporal lobe structures; it is 'a biological artifact of the human brain' (Persinger, 1987, p. 17).

Others, however, are more cautious and accurate in the statements they make about the role of the brain in religious experience. Newberg and d'Aquili clearly point out that their research says nothing about the existence of God. The findings do not mean that God is merely a bunch of brain cells firing. Nor do the results provide any kind of proof that God does exist. Like other scientific findings, when properly understood, this research says nothing about a philosophical position or matter of faith. The results have no implication for the reality of God. Of course, if we are to experience God, we must do so through our brains. What other organ would we use? But this is true for all of our experiences. As you read the words on this page, you are using your brain. As you listen to music playing over an iPod, you are using your brain. As mentioned earlier in the chapter, all of our experiences (thinking, feeling, believing, moving and so on) are mediated via the brain. The same must be true for religious experiences as well. This fact does not negate the validity of the religious experience any more than saying that enjoying a performance in a theater or symphony hall negates the validity of those experiences. We interact with reality by having that reality represented in our brains in the form of neural activity. While there is room for subjectivity in our interpretation of that reality, our 'neural story' nevertheless is considered by most scientists, and nonscientists as well, to be an accurate representation of the real world.

A leading figure in neuroscience and the integration of science and psychology is Malcolm Jeeves who suggests that we must understand a phenomenon from multiple levels (Jeeves, 2004b, pp. 28–30). The mental and the physical, for example, are different levels of a singular unity. These levels, however, are interdependent to Jeeves, and they form a duality of perspective, not a dualism of substance. Jeeves reports on a study by O'Craven and Kanwisher (2000) in which human subjects were asked to identify a visual picture. The pictures were either of houses or faces. While the subjects identified the pictures, brain imaging showed which areas of the brain became active. Different areas of the brain 'lit up' when the subjects looked at faces than when they looked at houses. Interestingly, the same areas became active when the subjects were asked to imagine in their mind's eye either houses or faces. In fact, the researchers could predict just by looking at the brain images what the subjects were thinking about or imagining, either houses or faces, because of the regular pattern of brain activation for the two kinds of objects. So is thinking about or imagining a face or house a mental or physical event? It is both, and can be considered from both a mental and a physical perspective.

It is in this way that we can speak of a religious experience as being both physical and spiritual. Yes, the brain is involved, just like it is involved when the O'Craven and Kanwisher subjects have a 'mental picture' of a house or face. So, too, the brain is involved when we have a 'spiritual or religious experience' such as praying. Both perspectives are valid and useful in trying to understand a complex human experience.

While we can view religious experience from different levels or perspectives, we should not make the mistake of thinking we have explained away any experience by identifying physical processes associated with the event. It is often said that religious experience, like most human experience, is irreducible or 'nonreductive' (Looy, Reimer and Seybold, 2005). Of course the brain (the body) will be affected and show changes when we have a religious experience. From a multiple levels perspective, however, that same religious experience can be understood from other objective and subjective viewpoints (see Chapter 4).

So was the experience I described at the beginning of this chapter religious or spiritual? Yes. It was also a physical experience that involved my brain and my entire body. Did God touch me is some special way that morning during worship? I believe he did. He touched me, however, through my physical being. I am an embodied child of God. I have a relationship with God through my embodied or physical nature. What it means to be an embodied creature made in the image of God is the subject of the next chapter.

Chapter 7

The Self

Terri Schiavo was 26 years old when she suffered severe brain damage due to insufficient oxygen reaching her brain. Over the next fifteen years, the American woman existed in a persistent vegetative state (PVS), a condition of unconsciousness in which the patient shows neither voluntary nor cognitive behavior, and which is considered by most neurologists to be irreversible. She was unable to communicate or even to eat on her own. A feeding tube supplied the nutrients that helped keep her alive. Terri's husband petitioned the courts in the state of Florida (where they lived) to remove the feeding tube on the grounds that it was not Terri's wish to live under the kind of circumstances brought about by the PVS. Her parents fought the husband in court (and in the media) to try to keep their daughter alive, even volunteering to assume responsibility for her care. Eventually, after a number of appeals, months of hearings, and involvement of the United States Congress, the courts decided that it was Terri's wish, as indicated by her husband, not to be kept alive under the conditions of the PVS. Her feeding tube was removed, and she died 13 days later on 31 March 2005.

Terri Schiavo's case polarized people in the United States, and elicited comments and pronouncements from politicians, ethicists and theologians. Even Pope John Paul II weighed in on the case. At stake, as one side saw it, was the right to life, no matter what kind of life it may be. Those who fought to keep Terri alive rejected the notion that Terri's condition was PVS, was permanent, or that she did not have any cognitive ability. They argued, among other things, that Terri did respond to those around her, and even showed signs of communication with her family and friends. Those on the other side believed that Terri would never return to even a shadow of her former self. They argued that her wishes should be followed, and that she should be allowed to die a peaceful death.

Also at issue in the Terri Schiavo case was the question of whether 'Terri Schiavo' still existed, even though her body was certainly alive. While perhaps no one stated the matter is such terms, nevertheless, part of the underlying tragedy concerned when a 'person' is no longer a 'person'. Similar questions arise in disease states like Alzheimer's (AD). While the exact causes of AD are uncertain, it is known that the brains of its victims show signs of abnormality such as plaques, tangles and cell loss. These abnormalities are thought to result in the memory problems so typical of AD and of the more severe cognitive changes found in the latter stages of the disease. In many respects, a person with AD ceases to exist. That is to say, the man with the disease is no longer the father his family once knew. Family members might think, 'This man is not Dad. Dad, as I remember him, is gone.'

These and other instances of neurological diseases and examples of brain damage raise important questions. Who am I as a person? What makes me the individual that I am? What makes me a unique 'self'? These examples even raise important questions about the nature of the soul. What is the soul? If personality and character can change so dramatically as the result of changes in the brain, to what extent is the essence of who we are as selves or souls connected to our brains? To answer these questions, we need to look at various ways of describing the self, the individual, the person that have been used in the past. We also need to consider the role of the mind in these issues, and how the mind and brain are related.

The Need for a Mind

As philosophers and early 'scientists' considered human nature and behavior, it became obvious to them that humans had certain abilities that animals did not share. Humans could think, they could reason, they could use language, and they had consciousness. Until the seventeenth century, there was no good way to explain these kinds of abilities except to postulate that humans had some special substance that animals and the rest of creation did not share. This special substance was called 'soul' by the early Greek thinkers. For Plato, the body and soul were two different kinds of things or substances. The soul was an immaterial thing; the body was a physical, material entity. Not only were the body and soul made of different kinds of stuff, the soul to Plato was eternal; it existed in the world of the Forms before occupying (or being imprisoned in) the mortal body at birth. As a result, the soul contained knowledge of the Forms which, to Plato, was true knowledge and ultimate truth. The soul also survived the death of the mortal body, returning to the world of the Forms.

The dualism of Plato was modified and Christianized by the early Church philosopher Augustine. Augustine's dualism saw the soul as immortal (rather than eternal), using a physical body (instead of being imprisoned in the body). Nevertheless, for both Plato and Augustine the soul represents the essence of one's personhood. Who we are as individual selves is tied to our immaterial souls. In dualism, the body is ultimately not important in who we are, because our identities survive the death of our bodies. The immaterial soul returns to the world of the Forms (Plato) or goes to God (Augustine).

Christian thinking about the self and personhood has traditionally included some form of dualism. The soul is considered to be the part of the individual that enjoys eternal life in heaven. The soul is that part of the individual that enables thought, reason, consciousness, memory and so on, and these qualities of humanness are those that continue in the afterlife with God. In the seventeenth century, René Descartes made a clear distinction between body and soul. The body was a machine to Descartes, and operated according to the laws of physics that were being discovered at that time. Animals were also machines, and could be understood according to physical laws. Humans, however, in addition to the material body, had an immaterial or non-physical soul which could not be described or explained through physics. It is the soul that makes humans different from animals, and it is the soul that enables rational thought, language and other human qualities. Because these human characteristics could not be explained by referring to physics, they required different laws and explanations. Nevertheless, according to Descartes, the immaterial soul interacts with the material body, and this interaction took place in a specific part of the brain called the pineal gland. The reason Descartes chose the pineal gland as the 'seat of the soul' and the point of interaction is because the pineal gland is singular: there is only one in the brain rather than one each hemisphere. Because consciousness in a singular phenomenon, Descartes reasoned that the soul had to be housed in a singular structure, not one that was divided into two different parts. Also, the pineal gland is in the center of the brain, perfectly located to control the physical body. Finally, some argue that Descartes selected the pineal gland as the location for the soul because of his incorrect belief that only humans had pineal glands. Because only humans (and not animals) had a soul, it made sense to locate the soul in a uniquely human brain structure. We now know that animals have pineal glands too, and many historians of science argue that Descartes, being familiar with general animal anatomy, would have known that as well. Regardless, it was the pineal gland that was the point of contact between the immaterial soul (the essence of personhood) and the material body.

By Descartes's time, the terms 'soul' and 'mind' were being used interchangeably. The mind was an immaterial substance separated from the physical or material body, and it was increasingly becoming the term used to describe what makes humans different from animals. The mind was the immaterial essence of what it meant to be a human being, the substance that enabled reason, thinking and language. Despite this change in terminology, much Christian thinking about the soul adopted the dualism of Plato, Augustine and even Descartes. The essence of who we are as people made in the image of God is our soul, and it is the soul (or mind) that enables us to function as human persons using the unique human characteristics of rational thought, language, consciousness and other qualities. Dualism seemed necessary for Christianity if there was to be any hope of eternal life. Obviously, the physical body dies and returns to dust; the soul, however, is not physical, and leaves the body at death. Because it is the soul that contains who we are as individual persons, the soul experiences either eternal reward in heaven or eternal punishment in hell.

Dualism, however, has a major problem. How can a nonphysical soul (or mind) affect the physical body? It seems obvious that the mind can and does affect the body, but how can this be accomplished if the body and mind are of two different substances, which is required in dualism? One of the accepted laws of physics refers to the conservation of energy, which says that energy cannot be created out of nothing. Energy can be changed from one form to another, but it cannot be created or destroyed. So how can the physical body be moved (a process that requires energy) by a mind that is not part of the physical world (and has no physical energy)? Dualism has never been able to account for this basic dilemma.

Today, the discussion of mind–body relationship takes a slightly different form. Instead of studying the relationship between mind (or soul) and body, philosophers and scientists talk about the relationship between the mind and the brain. In this more modern rendering of the millennia-old problem, how a mind that is considered to be immaterial can influence the physical brain is still the primary sticking point for dualism. Nevertheless, dualism still has its proponents, both in science and in philosophy (Goetz, 2005; Popper and Eccles, 1981).

Contemporary Alternatives to Dualism

The inability of dualism to explain how an immaterial substance (be it a mind or a soul) can affect a physical thing like the body has produced several nondualistic perspectives of this fundamental problem. One alternative is to see the mind as an 'epiphenomenon', a thing that 'goes along' with the body but has no ability to affect it. Much like a shadow 'goes along' with the body but has no ability to influence the body, the mind is such a phenomenon. Obviously, however, the mind does appear to really affect what the body does; it is not like a shadow, powerless over the actions of the body. Such a position, while proposed by some, is not a position that is widely accepted.

A second alternative to dualism is monism, the view that there is only one kind of thing, which is physical. There are a variety of forms of monism, including eliminative monism, the position that one can simply eliminate any discussion of mind because the mind does not exist. According to eliminative monism, there is only brain. Mind is a historical concept, one that has been shown to be unnecessary by contemporary neuroscience. As a result, any discussion of 'mental' can be reduced to brain activity. The mind *is* the brain. A particular type of mental state is identical to a particular type of brain state, and once that brain state is known, nothing remains to be discovered. Science can demonstrate that the brain is necessary for mental events such as consciousness, thought, language and reason to occur. Because of the necessary involvement of the brain, it is a short step to conclude that the mind is what the brain does; it is the brain in action, and nothing more. This last phrase, 'nothing more', is important. The late neuroscientist Donald MacKay warned scientists about 'nothing buttery' – the belief that once science provides a physical account of some phenomenon (such as mental activity), the phenomenon has been completely explained and nothing more remains to be uncovered or understood (MacKay, 1974). This form of monism is the position taken by many philosophers and scientists today, and is a natural outcome of the philosophical view known as reductionism. (See Chapter 4 for a distinction between philosophical or ontological reductionism and methodological reductionism.) The philosophers Daniel Dennett, Paul Churchland and Patricia Churchland, as well as scientists such as Francis Crick and Steven Pinker, are adherents to a monism that leaves no room for any discussion of mind.

Another kind of monism proposes that while the brain is clearly necessary for mental states to occur, a particular mental state is not identical to a particular brain state. Yes, some brain state must exist for the mental event to occur, but no particular brain state can be mapped onto the specific mental event in a one-to-one manner. This view of the mind–brain relationship avoids the dangers of reductionism inherent in eliminative monism (that is, the mind is nothing but the brain) and allows for the possibility of new properties (mental) emerging out of a physical substance (brain).

Reasons for Linking Mind to Brain

As indicated above, the mind was proposed to help explain the existence of certain human abilities such as reason, thinking and language. There was no known way that these qualities of human life could be explained physiologically, so a 'mental' explanation was offered. With the development of neuroscience in the twentieth century, but particularly during the last quarter of the century, the brain's role in these 'mental' abilities was clarified. Brain areas involved in language, thinking, reasoning and so on were identified, and a clear distinction between what is mental and what is physical became less defensible. One example of this is the research of O'Craven and Kanwisher (2000), who showed that the same brain area (a region of the ventromedial cortex) is active when we look at a physical object (such as a picture of a house) or create a mental picture of that object. Likewise, the ventral occipito-temporal cortex is activated when we look at an actual human face or when we imagine that person's face 'in our minds'. The researchers were ultimately able to predict, just by analyzing the brain scans, whether the subjects in the study were creating a mental image of a face (or house), or looking at a physical face (or house). So, given this kind of result, is thinking about the face of your grandmother a mental or physical event? The same brain area is activated in either case, so it seems that the act of thinking about your grandmother's face is best described as both a mental and physical event. Yes, the 'mental image' is created, but at the same time the brain is activated in the same area (although to a less intense degree) as it is when we are physically looking at our grandmother. What is mental and what is physical become very closely connected, leading the eliminative monists (or eliminative materialists) to do away with the mind altogether and just talk about the brain.

Other studies have shown similar close connections between brain activity and memory, decision making, forgiveness and even moral judgments. Greene and his colleagues, for example, found that certain brain areas are involved in making particular kinds of judgments (Greene et al., 2001). Using what are known as ethical dilemmas, the researchers found that personal moral judgments differ from nonpersonal moral judgments and other kinds of nonmoral decisions that people make, in that the personal moral judgments engage the individual's emotions in ways that other decision making does not. One such ethical dilemma involves a story in which a runaway trolley threatens the lives of five people. The only way to save the lives of these people is to redirect the trolley onto another track where a single person will be killed. You, the reader of the dilemma, are the only person who can throw the switch and change the trolley's course. Should you throw the switch? If you do, one person will die; if you do not, five people will be killed.

This dilemma is contrasted with a second, where again a trolley threatens the lives of five people. Now, however, you can only save the five individuals by pushing a stranger onto the tracks. The trolley will hit and kill the stranger, but in doing so will also be stopped, saving the lives of the other people. Should you push the stranger onto the tracks? Again, if you do not, five people will be killed; if you do, the five will be saved, but at the cost of the stranger's life.

Both dilemmas are similar in the number of lives saved and the number of lives lost. They differ, however, in one important aspect. In the first dilemma, you the reader must throw a switch to redirect the trolley. In the second, you the reader must perform a much more personal act. You must physically push another human being onto the track. Is one act more morally acceptable than the other? Most subjects given these dilemmas decide that it is morally acceptable to redirect the trolley, killing the single person but saving the five. However, the majority also believe that it is morally unacceptable to push the stranger onto the track to save the five people. Psychologically, the authors argue, the difference is in the degree to which the second dilemma engages the reader emotionally. Pushing a person to his or her death is considered a more personal and emotional act than turning a switch to redirect a train.

When the brains of the readers of these dilemmas were scanned using functional magnetic resonance imaging (fMRI), differences did appear. When reading the 'moral-personal' dilemma, areas of the brain involved in emotional processing did indeed become active. Reading the 'moral-impersonal' dilemma (pulling the trolley switch) failed to activate the emotional areas in the brain (or did so to a much lesser extent). The authors contend that the moral decision making in these kinds of dilemmas is accomplished, in part, by making use of the emotional processing occurring in the brain. Some moral decisions engage the emotional processing areas in the brain; others do not, or do so to a lesser degree. It is the activation of these brain areas (a physical event), therefore, that affects moral decision making.

Farrow and colleagues (2001) used fMRI to identify areas of the brain involved in empathy and forgiveness, while numerous researchers have investigated the brain areas involved in memory. These studies clearly show that the brain is involved in these 'mental' activities, and like the O'Craven and Kanwisher study, challenge a definite distinction between what is mental and what is physical.

Nonreductive Physicalism

Eliminative monists prefer to dispense with all talk of mind. Brain is all that exists; mind is a superfluous concept. Other monist perspectives, however, are less willing to jettison talk of the mind. While recognizing the close connection between mind and brain, proponents of these views suggest that the mind is dependent on the brain, but that it is a kind of emergent property of the physical brain. The concept of emergence sees the whole as being greater than the sum of its parts, and representing something completely and utterly new and different. The mind, as an emergent, depends on the physical brain, but is nevertheless a different property that cannot be viewed as consisting of nothing more that neurons and neurotransmitters.

A prominent view representing this kind of thinking is known as nonreductive physicalism (NRP), which accepts that the mind is dependent on the brain (that is, nothing nonphysical or immaterial is inserted into the brain to permit mental activity such as thinking), but insists that the mind is more than just the physical brain, and thus cannot be reduced to basic neural elements such as neurons. This view is best represented in the work of Nancey Murphy and Warren Brown, both on the faculty at Fuller Theological Seminary. Wanting to avoid the problems associated with both dualistic and reductionistic perspectives of the mind–body relationship, NRP is an attempt to integrate current findings from the neurosciences into an understanding of human nature that is true to the biblical story (Brown, Murphy and Malony, 1998; Murphy, 2006).

Brains are very complex physical structures. As indicated in Chapter 1, the human brain contains over 100 billion neurons, each neuron having on average 10 000 synaptic connections. The brains of other animals tend to be less complex. As we move from rats and mice (animals often studied by neuroscientists and psychologists) to dogs, monkeys, apes and humans, the brains of these species become increasingly more complex. According to NRP, somewhere along the evolutionary progression the brain becomes complex enough to enable certain abilities or powers, such as thinking, memory and decision making – in other words, the kinds of skills typically considered to be mental abilities. A mind has emerged, and we see this new property in the way the animal's behavior is changed. It is important to emphasize that according to nonreductive physicalists such as Murphy and Brown, what emerges is not a new *substance*, but new *causal powers*. In this way (among others), nonreductive physicalism attempts to avoid the label of dualism and the corresponding problems associated with that perspective. It is also necessary to point out that from a nonreductive physicalist perspective, mental abilities (and personhood itself) are, in part, the result of brain functions, but are also influenced by social and cultural forces as well as by the working of God in our lives (Murphy, 2005, p. 116).

Along this evolutionary continuum, the mind also becomes increasingly complex. The level of memory, decision making and thinking (if one wants to call it thinking) present in rats and mice is clearly less well developed than in dogs, monkeys, apes and humans. Again, according to NRP, somewhere along this progression the mind becomes sufficiently complex that a new property emerges out of mind: the soul. Warren Brown refers to this new property as 'soulishness' and Nancey Murphy prefers not to talk about the soul as a noun, because neither of these individuals (Brown is a neuropsychologist and Murphy is a philosopher) believes in a separate 'thing' or substance called a soul. We possess qualities of soulishness instead of having an independent soul. The importance of these mental qualities is that they each contribute to relatedness, and it is this quality of relatedness that is essential to Brown's concept of soulishness. The level of complexity of mind necessary for soulishness to emerge is a mind with the capacity for language, episodic memory, a theory of mind, conscious top-down agency and future orientation (Brown, 1998). Each of these qualities is important for humans to enter into relationships, and the relationships Brown believes signify soulishness are (1) a relationship with oneself (intrasubjective), (2) a relationship with others (intersubjective), and (3) a relationship with God. Part of a biblical picture of the human being is to see the self as constructed in relationship with other selves. The Bible emphasizes interdependence among selves for human identity, and it is this communal emphasis that is one of the ways the biblical picture of humanity is in contrast to a secular Western view of personhood which emphasizes individuality (Palmer, 2005, p. 192). Relationality is also emphasized in the Christian doctrine of the *imago Dei*. Genesis affirms that humans are created according to or after the image of God, but what does that really mean? From a trinitarian perspective, God is not an immaterial substance; God is relationship between the Father, the Son and the Holy Spirit (Shults, 2005, pp. 41–65). God must be understood as three persons in relation, and the glory of God is about the glorification of those three persons (Shults, 2003, p. 240). If we are made in the image of God, we are understood as 'persons' in relational terms – relations to others, and to God.

While researchers have attempted to teach nonhuman animals language, there is general agreement that these attempts have, at least thus far, failed. No one doubts that nonhuman animals can and do communicate (with both conspecifics and, perhaps, members of other species); however, the kind of communication represented in these animals fails to reach the level of language as commonly understood. True language requires creativity, grammatical constructions and semanticity.

Creativity refers to the ability within a language to create a potentially infinite variety of new sequences of sentences out of a comparatively finite number of words. The average speaker of American English, for example, might have a vocabulary of around 50 000 words, yet the number of sentences that can be created out of this lexicon is potentially unlimited. The kinds of communication found in subhuman animals lack this vital component. Grammatical constructions include requirements about word order, use of articles, past tense, possessives and so on. There are limitations in the kind of grammar we can use in language. We cannot just put any six words together in any order we want. Specific rules exist and must be followed (even if we do not explicitly know what those rules are or cannot tell someone else what those rules are). Semanticity refers to the way in which we assign meaning to words.

Human language use seems unique in its power. That is to say, humans are able to use language in ways that other animals cannot. This power enables the human communicator to send ideas, feelings, beliefs and so on from one person to another, to discuss the past, present and future, and to preserve these ideas, feelings and memories in a permanent form. The communication of these ideas, feelings, memories, beliefs and so on from one individual to another (or others) is fundamental in the development of relationships.

Another key component of developing relationships with others is the formation of long-term memories, particularly what psychologists refer to as episodic or autobiographical memories. Memory is not a singular phenomenon, but is instead composed of several different kinds of information. At the most basic level, memory is divided into declarative and nondeclarative types. Declarative, or explicit, memory consists of information that we can convey or tell to another. It is composed of memories that we know we possess; we have conscious access to these memories. Nondeclarative, or implicit, memory is information to which we do not have conscious access. We cannot verbally share this information with another. An example of this kind of nondeclarative information is my memory of how to ride a bicycle. While I may not be able to verbally describe in a step-by-step manner the procedures involved in riding a bike, I nevertheless know how to ride one, and can demonstrate this knowledge easily. The same can be said for tying one's shoes: we may not be able to declare verbally this knowledge to someone else, but we can certainly show another how shoes are tied. Another example of nondeclarative memory would be behavior learned via classical conditioning, such as salivating at the sight of a lemon.

Declarative memory is further divided into semantic and episodic forms. Semantic memory consists of information such as facts and general knowledge, the kind of information one might learn in a formal learning setting. Most people know that 5 plus 5 equals 10, and that Washington, DC is the capital of the United States. This kind of knowledge is easily 'declared' to others. In addition, however, we possess information about our own individual lives, the episodes of our own existence. This information, too, can be 'declared' to others. We can remember and tell others about our wedding day or the circumstances surrounding our being told about the death of a parent. These memories are also part of the declarative memory system.

We know that there are these two separate systems (declarative and nondeclarative) because some people who develop amnesia have a loss of declarative but not nondeclarative memory. A well-known example is the individual known only as 'H.M.' who developed amnesia as a result of brain surgery which removed large sections of his hippocampus, amygdala and related temporal lobe structures. As a result of this surgery and brain loss, H.M. lost the ability to form new declarative memories. Memories for events and general knowledge acquired prior to the surgery remained intact, but no new declarative memories were formed after the operation. A similar case is that of Clive Wearing, who experienced damage to similar temporal lobe structures as a result of Herpes Simplex Encephalitis, a viral infection of the brain. Clive Wearing also could not form new declarative memories. Nondeclarative memories, however, were intact for both H.M. and Clive Wearing. The temporal lobe structures lost in H.M. and Clive Wearing subserve declarative, but not nondeclarative memories. For a person suffering from this kind of amnesia, life consists of a series of moment-to-moment experiences. Any conversation held, any new person met, any information learned is quickly forgotten. While a person might remember vividly their wedding (if it occurred prior to the brain damage), they would not know or remember that their spouse died if that death happened after the damage to the brain occurred. For all intents and purposes, their episodic memory, in many respects their life as an individual person, stops when the brain is damaged.

Obviously, this kind of amnesia or failure of episodic memory can severely affect our relationships to others. We use our shared episodic memories to help develop relationships, be it with family members or friends. Without the ability to form new memories of what happens to us and others, we lose the ability to effectively relate to others. Without memory of what someone told us ten minutes ago, even casual conversations become nearly impossible.

A third mental ability that emerges with an increasingly complex brain is Theory of Mind (TOM), which is what psychologists call the ability to correctly attribute mental states to others. The ability to understand what another person might be feeling, thinking or believing are examples of TOM information that is available to an organism with a highly complex brain. Without this TOM knowledge, we cannot recognize that a person is upset at us, so we might say something insulting as a result. With a TOM, we see that the person we are talking to, perhaps our spouse, is already mad at us, and we avoid, if we are smart, saying something that will make our spouse madder still. While being inappropriate to our spouse might result in a temporary state of marital unrest, saying something inappropriate to our boss or a person who has obvious physical advantages over us might result in more permanent (perhaps bodily) harm.

TOM is also necessary for the development of healthy relationships with others. Empathy is an important ingredient in friendships. Being able to 'understand where a person is coming from' goes a long way in furthering relationships with others. So, too, is the ability to control one's behavior fundamental in forming relationships. This control is referred to as 'conscious top-down agency' by Brown (1998). With a sufficiently complex brain, the ability to modify behavior in a particular direction emerges. Animals with this capacity are not merely responding reflexively; intent is seen in behavior, and this intent is vital in forming relationships with others. An additional ability necessary to develop relationships is to have a future orientation – to be able to anticipate the consequences of one's behavior. Without such an orientation or without control over one's behavior, relationships with others would be unlikely because we would be constantly behaving in ways that might be pleasing to us, but would be unpleasant or even harmful to others. Psychologists call this kind of individual who cares for no one but his or her self an antisocial personality. Clearly, relationships with a person who has an antisocial personality are difficult if not impossible to maintain.

These qualities of mind emerge, according to Brown, in a brain that has reached a high level of complexity, and they enable the organism to develop relationships with others. These mental abilities are not limited to humans. While true language in nonhumans is unlikely, TOM, future orientation, top-down agency and episodic memory have been identified (to various degrees) in subhuman animals. However, these abilities seem to reach their fullest expression in humans, and it is in humans, says Brown, that the emergent mind develops sufficiently in complexity to allow for the emergence of what traditionally has been called the soul. It is in humans that these mental abilities allow for the development of relationships with ourselves, with others, and with God.

So the soul (or soulishness, as Brown prefers to call this uniquely human ability) is an emergent property of the mind, which is an emergent property of the physical brain. The mind and the soul are based on physical elements (the brain), but cannot be reduced to just the brain. The suggestion that the soul emerges from the mind which emerges from the brain implies that the mind, and ultimately the soul, cannot be completely explained by reference to brain activity and physical properties. There is more to soulishness than brain, and that 'more' is different than the brain. Not only is the whole greater than the sum of its parts, that whole is utterly new and different in important qualities and properties, ultimately unexplainable by reference to the parts. An analogy that is often used is that of hydrogen and oxygen. One can know all there is to know about hydrogen and oxygen as individual elements. However, nothing about hydrogen and oxygen would predict the wetness of water when these elements are joined. A new property emerges with the union of hydrogen and oxygen. In a similar manner, a new property emerges when the physical brain reaches a critical level of complexity. First, mental properties emerge, and then, with additional complexity, soulish properties emerge. It is these soulish properties that allow for personal relatedness, including our developing relationships with others and with God.

An essential question for a Christian is whether a particular idea, such as nonreductive physicalism, is consistent with biblical teaching. It very well might be the case that evidence from neuroscience and psychology suggests that personhood is based on our physical nature (our brains). Perhaps philosophers (such as Nancey Murphy) believe that the soul does not exist except as an emergent property from the brain. For a Christian, however, these philosophical or scientific ideas and findings need to coincide in a meaningful way with what scripture tells us about who we are as persons, who we are as creatures made in the image of God.

Fortunately, the evidence coming from neuroscience and psychology suggesting a physical basis for our personhood and identity (our soul) is consistent with the message presented by the Bible. Biblical scholars tell us that the Hebrew Scriptures point to a unity of personhood, not a dualism (Green, 2004a). The Old Testament does not teach that we are physical bodies plus an immaterial substance called a soul. The Old Testament also does not teach, according to these scholars, that our souls are independent of our bodies and that these disembodied souls survive the death of the body. We are unities or wholes. It is more correct to say that the Bible teaches that we *are* souls, not that we *have* souls. Not only does the Old Testament affirm the unity of personhood, so does the New Testament. The writings of Paul, for example, often taken to support a dualism in human nature, can be interpreted as reaffirming the unity of persons taught in the Hebrew Scriptures. 1 Corinthians 15 concerns the resurrection and the nature of the resurrection body, and in this discussion Paul refers to the 'physical body' which exists during this life on earth, and the 'spiritual body' which exists during the life following the resurrection (RSV). In the Greek, however, these terms refer to a body, provided by God, well suited to this age, and a body, also provided by God, well suited to the age to come. The current body is made of stuff of the earth and is perishable, dishonorable and weak. The post-resurrection body is made of heavenly stuff and is imperishable, honorable and powerful. The heavenly body is not an immaterial, ghost-like, disembodied 'spirit'. It is instead a body with characteristics that are appropriate for life in God's presence (Green, 2004b, pp. 97–8).

Embodied Souls

Doesn't the Bible teach dualism? Isn't the Bible clear that we have material bodies that die, but immaterial souls that live in eternity? Actually, the Bible teaches that we as human beings are physical things, and that what we call a soul is not an immaterial thing at all, but is a part of our physicality. We are embodied souls.

The key verse here is Genesis 2:7, which reads in the Revised Standard Version (RSV): 'Then the Lord God formed man of dust from the ground, and breathed into his nostrils the breath of life; and man became a living being.' 'Living being' is translated as 'living soul' in the King James Version. Three key points are present in this passage. First, God created man from the dust of the earth. Man is from the earth. Genesis 1 tells us that God commands the earth to 'put forth' vegetation and plants (Genesis 1:11) and the waters to 'bring forth' living creatures (Genesis 1:20). In Genesis 1:24, God tells the earth to 'bring forth living creatures according to their kinds' (RSV). Man is created out of the earth, out of the same kind of 'stuff' that is used to create the beasts of the field and the birds of the air (Genesis 2:19). Man and the animals have a common origin; man is linked with the rest of creation. In this respect, man is not a special creation; there is continuity between man, animals and all of God's creation. Lawson Stone argues that God did not cause the animals (including man) to form out of thin air. Instead, God instilled in what he made a part of his own creative action (Stone, 2004). The dust of the earth is able to 'bring forth' animals and ultimately man because of the creative act of God in the beginning. God provided what Howard van Till calls an 'optimally gifted' or 'fully gifted' creation, a creation that is able to 'bring forth' God's purpose and plan (Van Till, 2001, pp. 507–11).

Some might say that man is from the dust of the earth, but God provided the breath of life for man, and it is this breath of life that makes man special and different from the animals. The Hebrew word for 'breath of life' is also used to describe the animals, however. In the story of Noah, we read that God intends to destroy 'all flesh in which is the breath of life' by a flood (Genesis 6:17, RSV), and in Genesis 7:15 we read that 'two by two of all flesh in which there was the breath of life' went into the Ark with Noah. It seems that the Bible in these passages is telling us that this breath of life given to man by God was also given to the animals by God. It does not seem that this breath of life connotes an immaterial substance planted in man by God as a result of a special act of creation.

What happens when the breath of life is imparted? We are told in Genesis 2:7 that man became a 'living being' or a 'living soul'. Is this characteristic what makes man unique among creation? The Hebrew word used in this passage is *nefesh*, and it refers not to a separate part that is put into Adam, but to what Adam becomes or to what he is. Man does not have a *nefesh*. Man is a living *nefesh*. Man is a living being or soul. *Nefesh* is the inner core of each creature; it is what gives that creature, including man, its identity. Old Testament scholar Lawson Stone writes: 'No exegetical justification exists for finding here the notion of abstract, immortal, disembodied personhood that we usually mean when we speak of the "soul"' (Stone, 2004, p. 59). Thus, it seems that the research coming from psychology and neuroscience on the nature of who we are as persons is consistent with a biblical picture of human identity and the soul, at least the picture emerging out of the first few chapters of Genesis.

Support from Neuroscience and Psychology

Antonio Damasio is a researcher and neurologist at the University of Iowa and has spent many years working out an understanding of how the body (including the brain) helps create the mind and the self. For a sense of self to exist, not only must many brain systems be operational, but several whole body systems must be in full functioning mode. The self is created by neural systems that receive continuous input about the state of the entire body. This continuous updating of the body's condition is an important ingredient in the first of two sets of representations necessary for the neural basis of the self.

The first set of representations produces what Damasio calls the 'core self', which is a representation of the body generated by various brain structures (for example, the hypothalamus and basal forebrain) that are constantly being modified by updated input. At the same time, the brain is constantly sending neural and chemical information back into the body proper, further changing the body and continuing the evolving development of the body representation made by the brain (Damasio, 1994, p. 228). This continual updating of the current state of the body produces a rudimentary sense of the self that exists as long as there is input going to the brain from the body. Beyond this core self, however, is what Damasio calls the 'autobiographical self', which consists of representations of important events, facts, relationships, preferences and so on in a person's life. These long-term representations are made possible by the vast memory capabilities that humans enjoy and which are produced through the activity of brain structures in the temporal, parietal and frontal lobes. An important part of who we are includes our memory of who we were yesterday, who are the important people in our lives, what are the major events that have happened to us, what do we like and dislike, what are our values and beliefs, and many other such examples of information that help to define who we are as individuals. When we wake up in the morning, these two sets of representations instantly create a sense of self for us, a sense of self that is consistent with the identity that was present when we went to sleep the night before. So, despite the fact that our sense of identity and self 'goes away' while we are asleep (except for its appearance in our dreams – we recognize our selves in our own dreams, it is 'us' who is dreaming), it instantly re-emerges when we awake. This is made possible by the neural mechanisms, including input from the body as a whole, that constitute the core and autobiographical selves (Damasio, 1999, pp. 172–3).

Disorders that Affect the Self

'Personhood', 'identity', 'self' and 'soul' are terms we might use to name those special traits and characteristics that seem to separate us humans from the rest of God's creation. Terri Schiavo's case illustrates how the physical body, the brain in particular, is involved in creating who we are as human beings. When the brain is severely damaged, as was Terri Schiavo's, there can be a tragic but clear change in the ability of the individual to relate to others and to show signs of their former self. Most medical experts who examined Ms Schiavo diagnosed her condition as a persistent vegetative state, which is the diagnosis given to the most impaired patients with Traumatic Brain Injury (TBI). TBI deficits can range from mild to severe, and about 20 out of 100 000 people will die from TBI each year (Cummings and Mega, 2003, p. 394). Central nervous system syndromes associated with TBI include seizures, hydrocephalus, depression, psychosis and anxiety, to name just a few. The most severe of the syndromes is persistent vegetative state, which is characterized by wakefulness without alertness, a relatively normal sleep/wake cycle, nonpurposeful eye movements, spastic limbs, pain responses (for example, facial grimacing) and grasp reflexes, but no meaningful emotional or cognitive responses. It is important to know that to the neurologist, wakefulness is not the same thing as consciousness, and the person in a persistent vegetative state shows no evidence of being conscious (Damasio, 1999, p. 238). Physiologically, there can be a 60 percent reduction in glucose metabolism by the brain. Anatomically, there is cortical shrinking and demyelination (loss of insulation surrounding the neurons) throughout the cerebral hemispheres (Cummings and Mega, 2003, p. 396). Prognosis for recovery from persistent vegetative state is poor, particularly in a person in such a state for several years, as was Terri Schiavo.

A condition that might, on the surface, resemble persistent vegetative state is what neurologists call 'locked-in syndrome'. While the superficial symptoms might look like a vegetative state, the reality as far as consciousness is concerned is completely different (Damasio, 1999, p. 242). With locked-in syndrome, the individual has also experienced damage to the brain. However, the site of the damage is sufficiently different to have dramatic effects on the individual's state of consciousness and self-identity. The person with locked-in syndrome typically, and very suddenly, loses the ability to speak and almost all muscle movement; these losses are permanent. In this condition, however, the person is awake and fully conscious. It eventually becomes apparent that there are two movements the person can make: the person can move their eyes up and down, and the person can blink. The patient's entire diagnosis changes with those two small movements. In response to the right questions, the person can demonstrate with those movements that they are conscious of their surroundings, and can communicate that fact to medical personnel as well as family members. Sensations are intact, and the patient can understand what is going on around them. It is impossible, however, for the person to make any other kind of movement. This patient is fully aware of their environment. In addition, the identity or self of the person seems to be intact, as do the normal range of emotions, although there is a surprising lack of terror in the individuals given knowledge of their condition (Damasio, 1999, p. 292).

Both locked-in syndrome and persistent vegetative state are different from a coma, in which, again as a result of damage to the brain, the person appears to be asleep but no amount of stimulation will arouse them. Obviously, it is vital to correctly diagnose which condition a person has. Although coma, locked-in syndrome and vegetative state look similar in many ways, the effects on consciousness, identity and the self (especially between locked-in syndrome and vegetative state) are quite different.

Another neurological disorder that can affect identity and self is 'unilateral neglect', which can occur to individuals with damage (for example, due to a stroke) to the parietal lobe, especially in the right hemisphere. Of the two cerebral hemispheres, it is the right hemisphere, especially the prefrontal regions of the right hemisphere, which seems to be particularly involved in self-awareness and self-representation. Self-recognition, self-face/voice recognition, and first-person perspective each involve increased activity in the right hemisphere compared to the left, and self-related disorders, such as dissociative and depersonalized disorders which interrupt the unified sense of self identity, overwhelmingly involve damage to the right hemisphere (Kober et al., 2005, pp. 193–5).

Unilateral neglect is a disorder of spatial awareness and attention to stimuli contralateral to the site of brain damage. For example, if the damage occurs to the right side of the brain, the neglect will be for stimuli in the left visual or tactile field. There can be neglect to stimuli from the ipsilateral, or same, side as the brain damage, although this is a less frequent and less severe manifestation of the disorder (Heilman, Watson and Valenstein, 1993, p. 280). If the damage is severe (Mesulam, 2000, p. 194), the person may act as if half of the universe does not exist (for example, not be aware of the left side of visual space, personal space, the left half of the body and so on). For example, if asked to draw a picture of a daisy, a person with unilateral neglect might draw the flower without any petals on the left side. If asked to draw the face of a clock, all of the numbers for the hours will be jammed onto the right side of the clock. A man with neglect might fail to shave the left side of his face; a woman might fail to acknowledge her left arm, believing that the arm does not belong to her but to someone else. In each of these cases, the person is not suffering from mental disease (for example, delusions), but shows impairment in attention and/or recognition of spatial, visual, auditory or tactile stimuli. Explanations for the impairments seen in body image, self and identity include the hypothesis that the parietal lobes contain the neural mechanisms responsible for developing and maintaining a body schema, including the distinction each of us has between what is us (for example, our body), and what is not us (Heilman, Watson and Valenstein, 1993, p. 290). Because part of who we are, our identity and our self, is composed of our body schema, when the mechanisms responsible for building that schema are damaged, so is our sense of self, even to the point of not recognizing our selves as we should (for example, the man failing to shave the left side of his face). Chapter 6 on brain and religious experience discussed the research of Newberg and d'Aquili (2001, p. 4), where they found that inhibition of parietal lobe activity was associated with religious experiences in which the distinction between the self and the rest of the world was blurred. The experiences were reported as being close to God by Franciscan nuns, and as 'timelessness' or 'infinity' by Buddhist meditators. In neglect, of course, the seeming impairment of the self or identity is not temporary, but long-term, perhaps permanent.

Perhaps the best-known case of a change in identity or self is that of Phineas Gage, who suffered almost total destruction of his left frontal lobe as the result of a work-related accident in September of 1848. As described in more detail in Chapter 6, Gage miraculously survived the accident and lived another eleven years. There were, however, noticeable changes in his personality or identity. After the accident, Gage experienced a number of cognitive and intellectual changes, becoming irreverent, profane, impatient and impulsive, obstinate, and vacillating. The changes in the pre- and post-accident Gage were so profound that his friends reported that he was 'no longer Gage' (Macmillan, 2000, p. 93).

More familiar neurological disorders that seem to have an affect on one's identity and self include amnesia and Alzheimer's disease. Glenn Weaver reports on how identity and spirituality can be negatively affected in individuals suffering from these neurological conditions (Weaver, 2004, pp. 77–101). Amnesia, or memory loss, is a condition that not only affects the cognitive functions of learning and memory, but can also dramatically impair one's identity and how one relates to others. An example of this kind of impairment is anterograde amnesia, in which the person is unable to form new long-term memories. As discussed earlier, this kind of memory loss can be seen following damage to certain parts of the temporal lobe of the brain, especially the hippocampus. While memory for how to perform certain tasks (for example, drive a car or play a piano) remain intact, as do many memories that were created prior to the brain damage, the inability to form new memories impacts on what psychologists and memory researchers refer to as semantic and episodic memories. Semantic memories are of facts that we have learned and that we can declare or report to others (for example, the capital of the United States). Episodic memory (sometimes call autobiographical memory) consists of events in our lives that we can report to another person (for example, the details of one's high school or college graduation, events surrounding one's wedding day). When a person with temporal lobe damage loses the ability to form new semantic and episodic memories, it can result in a severe change in one's sense of identity and self. One well-known example of this kind of memory loss is that of Clive Wearing, who, as discussed above, suffered extensive bilateral damage to temporal lobe structures as a result of viral encephalitis. Wearing could no longer form any long-term memories about events in his life. So profound was the effect that he lost his memory of new events in his life within two minutes of the event's occurrence. He reported his experiences as being like an unconnected series of 'blinkered moments', and wrote in his diary several times during the day that he was 'now awake for the first time' (Weaver, 2004, p. 78).

Something of what it must be like to suddenly find yourself in the middle of some action or event in your life, but without any conscious knowledge of how you got into that situation, is portrayed in the Christopher Nolan movie *Memento* released in 2000. The movie is about a man, Leonard Shelby, who is injured during a murderous attack on his wife and can no longer form new long-term memories from the time of the attack onward. In his attempt to find his wife's killer, Leonard repeatedly and suddenly becomes conscious of his surroundings, but has no knowledge of where he is or why he is in that particular place. The audience gets a sense of what Leonard is experiencing through the fact that the scenes of the movie are shown in reverse order. So we, the audience, see Leonard find and kill the man he believes is his wife's murderer in the first scene of the movie, but we do not know who the people in the scene are or why one of them is killed. The next scene in the film shows what led up to the first scene, and in a similar manner we see the entire film last scene to first. As the scenes begin, the audience watching the film is constantly unsure of what is going on, just like real-life Clive Wearing must feel unsure of what is going on as he 'awakens to consciousness' multiple times during his day (Weaver, 2004, p. 78).

It is not too hard to imagine how one's sense of identity and self (not to mention ones' relationships with others) can be affected by such a neurological condition, an impairment produced by damage to particular structures of the brain.[1] When the long-term unity of experiences, beliefs and actions with which we are familiar and which

1 Other neurological disorders that can impair one's sense of self and one's interpersonal relationships can be found in books written by neurologists Todd Feinberg (2001), V.S. Ramachandran and Sandra Blakeslee (1998), and Oliver Sacks (1995, 1998).

is made possible through the working of our memory is disrupted, our sense of who we are as individual selves is impaired as well (Weaver, 2004, p. 85). This disruption in memory, and thus the identity, is produced when particular brain structures (for example, the hippocampus and other temporal lobe regions) are severely damaged. Similar structures (along with other areas of the brain not involved in amnesia) are damaged in Alzheimer's dementia, a condition that affects approximately four million people in the United States and 340 000 in the United Kingdom (Weaver, 2004, p. 81), or around 10 percent of all adults over the age of 65 (Knight, 1992, p. 129). Alzheimer's disease is a brain disorder characterized by amyloid plaques (a center of amyloid protein surrounded by scar-like tissue), neurofibrillary tangles (bundles of protein filaments inside the neuron), and cell loss in temporal-limbic structures and the frontal lobe cortex. The clinical presentation includes impairments in short- and long-term memory, judgment, abstract thinking and personality. In the latter stages of Alzheimer's disease, motor control and language can be lost. There is neither a cure nor effective treatment for Alzheimer's disease, and the time course from diagnosis to death is approximately eight to ten years on average.

How might a disease like Alzheimer's, particularly in its later stages, affect identity and self? Weaver interviewed 'partner observers' of Alzheimer's patients and found a number of perceived changes in identity and spiritual expression in the loved ones by these 'partner observers'. Observed changes included loss of the patient's spiritual life narrative, a sense of spiritual emptiness, diminished participation in spiritual practices (for example, personal prayer and corporate worship), difficulty experiencing God's comfort, and experienced guilt about the loss of close relationships in a community of faith (Weaver, 2004, p. 86). Disruption in memory (a hallmark symptom of Alzheimer's disease) and sense of agency impairs the patient's ability to read or listen to scripture, hear sermons or actively participate in worship. Of course, we do not question the 'spirituality' of the affected person just because they are suffering from a terrible disease and are not participating in private or corporate worship as they once did. It is important to note, however, that those patients who tended to rely on these kinds of activities in their spiritual practice often found it more difficult to feel close to God and benefit from his presence as a result of the disease, a time when they perhaps needed this kind of comfort the most (Weaver, 2004, p. 89). Despite the changes mentioned above, the partner observers continued, in many cases, to still see signs of spiritual vigor in their loved ones, as expressed in the relationships between the Alzheimer's patient and important figures in their lives. Weaver identifies a number of practical ways to facilitate the maintenance of these important interpersonal relationships, even as the disease progresses to its final stages. Thus, even though one's identity is physically embodied and the brain plays a critical role in the creation of 'the self', identity is also, in part, socially embodied, and it is that component of identity that can be assured by loved ones even as disease ravages the brain.

A final disorder that can affect the self is schizophrenia. Like the disorders already mentioned (amnesia, neglect, Alzheimer's), schizophrenia is a psychiatric disease that affects the brain. While the exact causes of schizophrenia are unknown, it is associated with significant damage to brain tissue, including temporal lobe structures and portions of the frontal lobe. It is disconnectivity within the frontal lobe, especially the prefrontal cortex (PFC), that seems most detrimental to the self and identity. Schizophrenia is characterized by both 'positive' symptoms (the abnormal presence of some class of behavior) and 'negative' symptoms (the absence of some behavior that is typically present and whose presence is considered to be normal). For example, delusions (false beliefs such as thought insertion or thought broadcast) and hallucinations are hallmark positive symptoms of schizophrenia. Negative symptoms include a flattening or absence of affect (emotion), psychomotor poverty and social withdrawal. Some have argued that the essential problem in schizophrenia is a 'disturbance of the self model or the "self-monitoring" capacity' of the individual (Vogeley et al., 1999, p. 343), and it is this 'self-monitoring' capacity in which the prefrontal cortex is especially important.

The PFC is an area of the frontal lobe where information from the major sensory regions of the brain (for example, vision, audition, touch, taste and smell) converges and is integrated. This integration is necessary to develop a coherent understanding or model of the world and the self's place in it. The parietal lobe (particularly in the right hemisphere) is crucial in creating this image of the body and its place in the external environment. Connections between the PFC and the parietal lobe enable the creation of a model of the person with his or her environment. Disconnection with the PFC impairs this self model, and contributes to many of the symptoms seen in schizophrenia that reflect impairment of this model, including thought broadcast or insertion (disturbance of ownership), hallucinations (failure to recognize self-induced internal perceptions) and disruption of a theory of mind, which could contribute to social withdrawal (Vogeley et al., 1999, p. 352). The PFC is part of the brain mechanism that generates experiences of ownership and unity of perspective, a mechanism not fully functional, it seems, in schizophrenics.

Implications for Christian Belief

> For I know that my Redeemer lives, and at last he will stand upon the earth; and after my skin has been thus destroyed, then from my flesh I shall see God, whom I shall see on my side, and my eyes shall behold, and not another. (Job 19:25–27a).

Views of human nature, personhood, the self and the soul are of more than merely theoretical interest. Such perspectives can have consequences on how we practice our Christian faith. Our understanding of the nature of personhood can affect how we treat others individuals, how we view the sacraments of baptism and the Eucharist, as well as our approach to Church ministry and personal evangelism.

For example, what is the role of the Church in its ministry to others? Is it to save souls for a better afterlife? Is it to show concern for personal suffering and social injustice in this life? Is it to become involved in political movements directed at relieving the physical distress of the people of the world? Is it to make sure the people of the Church are ready for the Second Coming of Christ and the Rapture? A critical assessment of dualistic views of personhood and the self might suggest that these approaches to human nature that emphasize the immaterial soul as the 'essential' part of one's identity tend to ignore the physical part of the person in an effort to save the soul. Ultimately, the critique suggests, dualism views the essential self as immaterial, and Christian dualists see the immaterial soul as what Christ died to save. Also, it is the immaterial soul that will spend eternity with God in heaven, so there really is no eternally important reason to be too concerned with physical conditions, social injustice or the affairs of this material world.

A physicalist perspective on personhood would not be criticized in this manner. To the physicalist, the body is vital for personhood. The physical state of the individual is something to be concerned about because the person is a biological-psychological-spiritual unity. There is no immaterial component to the self. There is no immaterial soul to save for eternity. So this perspective of human nature is more conducive to a view of Church ministry that emphasizes the physical, psychological as well as spiritual needs of the person. A critic of such a theory might argue that physicalists, even if they call themselves nonreductive physicalists as Brown and Murphy do, must make a stronger case than they have thus far for why physicalism is not, ultimately, nothing but a form of reductionism. If physicalism is essentially reductionism, then how is the Church anything more that just another kind of social agency addressing the physical needs of the person, since physical needs are all that really exist. So how we understand the nature of personhood (either from a dualistic, physicalist, or some other perspective) might influence how we carry out the work of the Church, what programs we create and fund, and what kind of services we provide for others.

Our view of who we are as persons can also influence how we approach and understand important rituals and sacraments of the Church, such as baptism and communion. In baptism, what is the role of the water? Is it to symbolize the cleansing of the immaterial soul, or of the entire person? In the Eucharist, we commemorate the suffering and death of Christ on the cross. We partake of his body and his blood (either symbolically or literally, depending on one's Church affiliation), reminding us that Christ sacrificed his whole self for the forgiveness of our sins. And speaking of forgiveness, how do we understand the purpose and result of granting or receiving forgiveness? A dualistic perspective might be criticized because by emphasizing the immaterial soul as the essential aspect of who we are as persons, it tends to ignore the physical nature of humanity and our physical relationships with others. If the essential me is really immaterial and nonphysical, then what is important in forgiveness is how my inner, immaterial self is changed. The physical part of who I am, because it is not ultimately important to the real me, need not be of any real concern. The physical relationships I have with others are also, ultimately, unimportant because those physical relationships cannot affect who I really am – a nonphysical, immaterial soul. On the other hand, if I am a physical-psychological-spiritual unity, then the physical side of me, including my physical relationships with others, will be vital in any kind of forgiveness that I might receive or grant. The Eucharist reminds us of the whole-person sacrifice of Jesus and the forgiveness he offers to us as whole-persons (biological, psychological and spiritual). So forgiveness needs to be understood as affecting my whole being. This is certainly consistent with the traditional Christian understanding of what forgiveness is, an understanding that does not come from a dualistic view of human nature, but from a more physicalist-holist perspective. As Stuart Palmer reminds us:

> It is never the case in the Christian tradition that one's soul receives forgiveness in a way that excludes one's bodily existence … Thus, a traditional understanding of forgiveness is not expressed with only parts of the person (i.e., the soul) or received with parts of the person

> (i.e., the body), but is intended to be holistic and embodied in expression and in reception. (Palmer, 2005, p. 207)

Perhaps the most obvious part of Christian faith that is affected by how one views human nature is the belief in life after death. It is widely held that an immaterial soul is necessary to make life after death possible. The immaterial soul, so the argument goes, does not need the body, and it is this immaterial soul that spends eternity with God; so the death of the physical body is not seen as a major obstacle to be overcome. On the other hand, a physicalist view of personhood holds that who we are is dependent, in some way, on our physical nature. We as persons and selves are not 'nothing but' our physical bodies, but without our physical bodies 'we' would not exist, either in this world or the next.

Biblical hope in eternal life should not be based, however, on a belief that an immaterial, purely spiritual soul survives outside of the physical body. Christian hope in eternal life is expressed well in the words of the Apostles' Creed: 'I believe in the resurrection of the body and the life everlasting.' As these words emphasize, it is a resurrected body that Christians believe in, not a disembodied, free-floating, immaterial soul. Can we really believe that our bodies will somehow be restored after the ravages of death and decomposition? Are we recreated with new physical bodies, or reassembled from molecules of our old body? There have been many attempts to address this important issue, none of which reach anything close to a consensus among theologians, philosophers or biblical scholars (see, for example, Corcoran, 2001; Green, 2004b, pp. 85–100). What is important to remember, however, is that the promise of resurrection comes not from science or philosophy, but from the revelation found in scripture. The nature of the resurrection is also found in scripture. As the passage in Job above suggests, from our flesh we shall see God; we shall behold him with our eyes (a physical act). Ted Peters, theologian at Pacific Lutheran Theological Seminary and the Graduate Theological Union, puts it this way:

> What is raised is the whole person inclusive of our various aspects: body, soul, and everything else. This does not forbid positing the existence of a human soul. What it forbids is the notion of a permanent disembodied soul that bears the essence of a person's identity. Theologically, it would be a mistake to think of our soul as our true person, thereby rendering the body an unnecessary appendage or a prison from which to seek escape. It would be a mistake to think of the soul as having a built-in capacity for immortality that can bypass the need for a divine act of resurrection. (Peters, 1999, p. 323)

If God can create me originally, in all of my physical, psychological, social and spiritual unified nature, then surely he can do so again in a resurrected body. Who I am, my identity, my self, is tied to my physical being, especially my brain. How can the person I am, dependent as I am on my physical existence, hope for eternal life with God? It is through the resurrection of my body, however God might accomplish it. This resurrection is a result of the grace of God. It is a divine act, promised in scripture, not guaranteed by philosophy or science. Ultimately, I guess, that promise will have to do.

Chapter 8

Evolutionary Psychology

One day as Jesus was teaching, a man asked Jesus what must be done to inherit eternal life. Jesus responded by asking the man what the law requires. Correctly, the man replied that the law says to 'love the Lord your God with all your heart, and with all your soul, and with all your strength, and with all your mind; and your neighbor as yourself'. When the man was told by Jesus to follow the law, he wanted to know who counted as a neighbor. In answer to this, Jesus told the story of a man who fell among robbers, was stripped, beaten and left for dead. Two people (a priest and a Levite) came upon the man, but did nothing to help. A third man, a Samaritan, saw the man and had compassion on him. He bandaged the injured man's wounds, took him to a nearby town and paid for his recovery. This famous story of the 'Good Samaritan' (Luke 10:25–37) tells us that we should treat all people as neighbors, even those who are our enemies and despise us. It also is a beautiful account of altruism, doing something good for another person with no expectation of having the good deed returned to you.

In the past, many cultures have imposed severe punishments, up to and including death, on women found guilty of adultery. The guilty man, however, was often not dealt with so severely. The adulterous act was seen as an offense against the husband of the woman, with the husband entitled to certain legal or financial compensation. In nineteenth-century France, if a husband whose wife had committed adultery exacted revenge against the guilty man, French law imposed a lesser penalty in recognition of the understandable anger that the adultery created in the offended husband (Barrett, Dunbar and Lycett, 2002, p. 182). In the biblical story of the woman caught in adultery (John 8:1–11) the scribes and Pharisees, following the law of Moses, wanted to stone the woman. No mention is made, however, of the man also caught in the illegal act. While these extreme punishments are less likely found in today's societies, there often continues to be a distinction between how an adulterous woman and an adulterous man are perceived and even treated by others. Why should adultery in a woman be considered worse than adultery in a man?

Men and women get married every day. They promise to love and cherish each other through sickness and health, wealth and poverty, until death separates them. Why would a man make such promises? Why would a woman? Are the reasons the same for each? What accounts for a male and a female forming such a marriage bond? There are several differences between men and women in the cost of sex and parenting, as well as the overall goal of propagating one's genes. Sex is relatively inexpensive for men; sperm are created by the millions, and the goal is to create as many offspring carrying your genes as possible. The cost of parenting is nearly zero for a man. He does not have to carry, give birth or feed the child. For a woman, on the other hand, the cost of sex and parenting is high. Eggs are relatively rare (only a few hundred during the course of a woman's lifetime), and the woman must bear, birth and care for the child that results from sexual intercourse. While the reasons for a woman wanting a 'mate' to help take care of the child are understandable, why would a man agree to such an arrangement? One account maintains that marriage was ordained by God. Eve was created by God so Adam would have a helper and friend, someone with whom Adam could share his life. A monogamous union between a man and a woman is God's wish and plan for humanity. Another account, however, considers the differences mentioned above between males and females, and develops an explanation of marriage based upon these distinctions. In addition, these variations between males and females are used to help explain why men are more promiscuous, more violent, more drawn to pornography, more jealous of sexual infidelity, and more easily sexually aroused than women, and why, when there is a large age difference between a couple, it is usually the man who is with a younger woman. This account makes for an interesting story, but is it true, and is it compatible with the biblical ideal developed in the story of Adam and Eve in the Garden of Eden?

Each of these subjects – altruism, differences in adultery, and monogamous relationships – is studied by a relatively new sub-area of psychology known as evolutionary psychology. Evolutionary psychology (EP) seeks to bring an evolutionary approach and understanding to human behavior. From this perspective, all behavior can ultimately be understood as the result of natural selection and adaptation (Barrett, Dunbar and Lycett, 2002, p. 1). The principles of evolutionary biology can also be used to understand the development and function of the human mind (Buller, 2005, p. 17). Indeed, evolutionary psychology is being touted by some as the new paradigm for psychological science, bringing the disparate fields of current psychology under the umbrella of an evolutionary worldview (Buss, 1995). According to these evolutionary psychologists, all areas of psychology, personality, perception, learning, development and cognition can be understood and explained by bringing an evolutionary viewpoint and Darwinian insights to the questions these sub-areas of psychology study (Gaulin and McBurney, 2004, p. 1).

Altruism

No area has received greater interest in EP than altruism, which can be defined as helping another at some risk to one's self. Altruism has received so much attention in EP because it seems to go against natural selection. Darwin's theory of evolution emphasized random variation of traits within nature which, when combined with a struggle for existence among individuals, produces natural selection (Miller, 1999, pp. 7–9). One only has to look at the great variety of dogs at a dog show to see how humans have created various breeds with a tremendous range of traits, selected by breeders for specific purposes and reasons. The same occurs in nature: a great variety of traits exists among individual organisms in the plant and animal kingdoms. All living things can reproduce, and there is a limit to the number of progeny that can survive. As a result, there will be a struggle among the individuals of a species for survival. Those individuals whose random traits (we now know that these traits are passed on to the next generation via genes) increase their adaptability to a particular environment will be more likely to survive than those whose random traits impair their adaptability. This is the process of natural selection, which acts automatically and results in the continuation of those traits, passed on to the next generation, which increase the adaptability, and therefore the survivability, of the individual members of the species. The process can also result, given enough time, in the creation of new species.

If the foundation of natural selection and evolutionary theory, upon which EP is based, is survival and the passing of one's genes to the next generation, why would an individual help another when the assistance puts the helper at some risk or danger of death, in other words decreasing the helper's survivability? Some biologists have defined altruism by suggesting that apparent acts of altruism are selfish in reality, because the helping behavior is only performed to make the altruist feel good, to increase the reproductive success of the altruist, or to increase the prevalence of altruistic genes in the gene pool (Barber, 2004, p. 9). Critics argue that this approach to altruism defines it out of existence, making the 'problem' of altruism go away for biology. Altruistic acts, however, do not go away that easily. There seem to be legitimate examples of altruism, both in animals and humans. Some examples, such as parenting, can be understood, at least in part, by explaining them in terms of promoting the genes of the parent. Other examples of altruism, for example food sharing and cooperation among members of a group, are more difficult to understand in terms of individual genetic survival. Such altruism is seen as a characteristic of groups and influenced by social context (Barber 2004, p. 10). What motivates a person to join the military and sacrifice personal welfare, even to death? Can this act be understood from an evolutionary perspective? Exactly how does the individual making the sacrifice benefit? How does the group or society benefit? Is the human tendency toward cooperation, and even conformity, an evolved trait? How does EP 'explain' such examples of altruism?

Altruism is seen in many species of insects, for example honeybees and wasps, which have developed an organized social structure, called 'eusociality' by biologists, which consists of various levels of workers, each performing specific tasks for the good of the hive. Some of these workers display altruism in that they do not reproduce themselves, so their genes do not get passed on to the next generation, but they continue to work for the larger group. This kind of altruism represents a major challenge to evolutionary theory, as Darwin himself admitted. However, when the genetic system of the species that display eusociality is considered, this form of altruism becomes less of a problem for evolutionary theory. In all but one species that demonstrates this kind of social scheme, the genetic system (called haplodiploidy) found is one in which an individual shares 75 percent of their genes with their sisters instead of the more typical 50 percent. In other words, they are more closely related genetically to their sisters than they would be to their own offspring. So working to ensure the survivability of one's sisters is actually more likely to result in the continuation of these workers' genes than if they had their own progeny. This process, known as kin-selection, supports an evolutionary account of altruism, even though what are being selected are not the individual's genes through their own offspring, but the individual's genes through their sisters and the sisters' offspring. Kin-selection is an example of a kind of 'selfish altruism' that biologists can handle with relative ease.

Kin-selection, however, cannot explain the form of altruism typically observed in human beings or in most of the animal kingdom. Many examples of altruism are seen between two individuals (or between an individual and a group) who are not closely related genetically. In an attempt to explain this brand of altruism, the term 'reciprocal altruism' has been used, and describes a situation where one individual does something helpful to another with the idea that the favor will eventually be returned. The phrase 'I'll scratch your back and you scratch mine' illustrates this kind of reciprocal behavior. EP argues that this altruism is also ultimately selfish, because the individual expects something positive in return, even if the positive payoff is a long time coming. (Critics of EP argue that this is an example of redefining altruism out of existence.) In addition, keeping track of who has helped who among a social group requires certain cognitive abilities, those abilities becoming increasingly more complex as the social group becomes bigger (Leahey and Harris, 2001, pp. 405–8). With reciprocal altruism comes the chance that cheating will occur, that is to say that a person who is helped will not return the favor and aid the altruistic person or help others who might be in need. EP suggests that cultural evolution has produced several institutions that enforce reciprocity within a society, including police, the law, and even religion. These institutions enforce the fundamental importance of reciprocity through rules, regulations, mores, conscience and the appeal to emotions such as guilt and shame. Individuals who ignore the rules, laws and guilt feelings run the risk of being ostracized from society. Ethical and moral behavior are seen as ways of helping to ensure that equality of social exchange is maintained in societies as they get larger, and that individuals who follow these behaviors remain included in the social matrix (Schloss, 2004, pp. 10–11).

Whether EP can explain altruistic acts such as joining the military or sacrificing one's life for another is questionable. There is a certain sense in which even these kinds of altruistic acts can be understood from a social group perspective. That is to say, as social groups become larger over the course of human history, from a small band of perhaps five individuals to bigger groups represented by tribes and clans, there remains some possibility of reciprocity. Perhaps the same tendencies exist today, and are played out in the even larger social group represented by a nation. EP might suggest that a person joining the military is making a sacrifice with the expectation of getting something from the nation (or the people of the nation) in return. As we will see with other behaviors that EP tries to explain, the 'story' EP creates might make a certain amount of intuitive sense; however, the empirical evidence to support that 'story' is for the most part lacking. That does not mean the EP story regarding altruism is false, just that it is based upon a lot of assumptions, speculation and guesswork.

Sexual Behavior, Monogamy and Parenting

The beginning point for an EP account of sexual behavior, monogamy and parenting is the difference between males and females in terms of mating opportunity and parental investment. In most species, it is the male that has to struggle for the opportunity to mate with a female. Not all males will get the chance to reproduce; almost all females will. In addition, the investment in parenting, particularly in humans, is much greater in the female than in the male. Females produce a limited number of eggs during the course of a lifetime, a few hundred at the most. It is the female who carries the child, who births the child, and who nurses the child. Each of these tasks requires a great deal of energy and, in the case of carrying and birthing the child, risk to health and even life. Also, compared to other species, human infants are born completely helpless, and remain in need of an adult's care for many years. A newborn deer might be able to fend for itself after only a few weeks of life, but obviously it will be several years before a human child will mature enough to become independent from its parent, and it is typically the female parent who bears the greater responsibility for the care of the child. (The point at which such independence is reached varies from culture to culture, but in all societies it is a multi-year process.) For the human male, however, the picture is dramatically different. Sperm are relatively cheap, in that they are produced by the millions, and males remain capable of producing sperm well into late adulthood. In addition, the male does not have to carry or give birth to the child. His parental responsibilities, in this regard, are insignificant.

According to EP, these differences in mate competition, cost of reproduction, and parenting responsibilities put different pressures on human males and females that are reflected in patterns of sexual behavior and parenting. Because sperm are so cheap and easy to reproduce, EP suggests that males are driven to have sexual intercourse with as many females as possible. Remember, the goal is to transfer one's genes to the next generation. For the male, the best way to do this is to impregnate as many females as possible, especially because he has, compared to the female, limited parenting duties. As mentioned above, however, not all males get the opportunity to mate, so there is great competition among males for females. Finally, males might be driven to impregnate as many females as possible and might have limited parenting responsibilities, but there is no way for a male to be certain of his paternity. According to EP, these characteristics are why males are more easily sexually aroused, are more promiscuous, are more aggressive and are more jealous of sexual infidelity than are females. Quick sexual arousal and promiscuity make sense because the goal is to impregnate as many females as possible. Limited supply of females contributes to the heightened aggression in males, and the lack of certainty about paternity makes males more jealous of sexual infidelity in their mates.

For the female, the picture painted by EP is different. She must select from all of the male suitors the one best able to give her strong, healthy children. In other words, the female is looking for the male who offers the best genes, and uses cues such as self-assurance and assertiveness as indicators of genetic fitness (Gangestad et al., 2004). According to EP, however, the woman, unlike the man, is not looking for a series of one-night stands. In addition to genetic fitness, she is looking for long-term stability in a relationship where the man will help her raise children to maturity. (Gangestad et al. (2004) found that while women who are ovulating prefer men who are assertive and self-assured, during low-fertility days the women did not prefer these qualities in males.) Because of these differences in parental investment and reproductive costs, the woman is less promiscuous, less easily sexually aroused and less physically aggressive than the male. In addition, this conflict between what women look for and what men want leads, according to an EP perspective, to a monogamous relationship between men and women. The man trades his sexual promiscuity for a monogamous relationship in which he is certain of his paternity, the knowledge that he is raising his own offspring. The woman, on the other hand, gets help in raising the children from the male in return for sexual exclusiveness with her husband.

In this kind of arrangement, EP makes certain predictions about family dynamics. For example, according to EP, males should be especially jealous of any suggestion of sexual unfaithfulness in their spouses. Females, on the other hand, will be jealous of sexual unfaithfulness, but they will be even more jealous of any outside relationship that threatens the long-term emotional relationship with their spouse (Buss et al., 1992; Buunk et al., 1996). The primary concern for the male is paternity, and any relationship by his spouse that challenges that paternity is a threat to the man. The female, on the other hand, is primarily concerned with maintaining a strong, committed relationship with her husband, and any outside relationship that potentially interrupts that emotional bond with her spouse is going to be seen as threatening. Sexual infidelity might pose a threat, but is more easily forgiven and understood than a developing emotional relationship with another woman, even if it is nonsexual.

These evolutionary pressures on males and females have certain implications for violence, particularly homicide. A preschool child who lives in a home with a step-parent is a hundred times more likely to be killed. Of course, the vast majority of step-parents do not harm their stepchildren, and the figure above can give a misleading picture of the nature of most relationships between children and their step-parents. Nevertheless, the largest homicide risk factor for preschool children is having a step-parent in the home (Buss and Duntley, 2003, p. 125), a fact that perhaps can be better understood if approached from an EP point of view. This viewpoint would also predict that a male, given his heightened jealousy of sexual infidelity in his mate, would be more likely than a female to harm that mate if a sexual indiscretion should occur. In fact, empirical evidence suggests that such sexual infidelities are the largest risk factor for a young woman being killed (Buss and Duntley, 2003, p. 126). Even rape is considered by some evolutionary psychologists as a 'natural' means by which men can get more of their genes passed to the next generation, an adaptive behavior that evolved due to the different sexual strategies used by men and women described above (Thornhill and Palmer, 2000, p. 84). This EP account of sexual mate selection, monogamy, male–female dynamics and parenting is not without its critics, who point out the tremendous flexibility or even contradictory nature of the overall perspective (a theory of everything), the excessive use of speculation in lieu of empirical evidence, and the questionable rigor of the science underlying the theory (Van Leeuwen, 2001).

When it comes to trying to understand sexual behavior, monogamy and parenting, EP paints a very interesting picture. There is a certain amount of coherence within the story. It tends to make sense; it seems to explain much of human behavior. There certainly are some empirical studies that support the hypotheses made by

EP regarding sexual behavior (for example, the research on differences in jealousy in men and women). As with altruism, however, the empirical evidence is not as extensive as EP theorists would like or as one is led to believe reading the EP literature, especially in books. It is for this reason that some critics of EP have called many of the explanations proposed by the theory 'just-so stories' (Gould, 2000, p. 119). EP argues it can explain why the human species is so aggressive (for example, competition for limited resources), but it also can explain why there are examples of nonaggressiveness among human beings (for example, reciprocal altruism and arranged alliances among competing social groups). An EP viewpoint is provided for why males of certain species do not have strong paternity instincts, but also for why males of other species do show strong paternal behaviors. A person reading the EP literature comes away with the impression that EP is trying to explain everything using an evolutionary perspective, and that no matter what the results of an experiment might yield, those results can be used to support an EP account (Van Leeuwen, 2001, p. 104). Too often, say the critics, these 'explanations' seem too perfect and neat, almost contrived.

Morality and Ethics

In addition to the topics discussed above, EP is also used to understand and explain moral and ethical behavior. Like the moral act of altruism, all moral and ethical behavior has the sole function of passing along genetic information, and any account of ethical or moral behavior must have a biological, or more specifically, an evolutionary basis. Can evolutionary theory really make any contribution to an understanding of the origin and content of ethical and moral systems? Are the mechanisms proposed by Darwin the best (only?) explanations for why one ethical pattern of behavior is selected over another? Why should any moral or ethical system (that is, an orientation to what is right or good, wrong or bad) exist at all (Schloss, 2004, p. 7)? These questions (and their answers) have important implications for traditional Christian beliefs about the source of moral law and the origin of evil.

One evolutionary account of morality and ethics is to see these behaviors as by-products of cognitive abilities that evolved to serve other, non-ethical, functions. For example, the cognitive abilities of being able to anticipate future consequences of one's behavior, assign a hedonic label (positive or negative) to the consequence, and to choose among possible behavioral outcomes are used or co-opted to make decisions regarding ethical and moral behavior. These abilities did not evolve in order that ethical decisions could be made. They evolved because individuals with these cognitive abilities had a survival advantage; however, the behaviors were also used by individuals to make decisions regarding what is ethical and moral.

Another account sees adaptation playing a more direct role in the evolution of ethical/moral behaviors. For example, an EP perspective on the almost universal taboo against incest might see this moral rule evolving in the following way. First, offspring of an incestuous relationship are more likely to suffer from various mental and/or physical disorders, so incest represents a threat to fitness and survival. Second, those individuals with an aversion or repulsion toward incest would be selected for (or the genes for those responses would be selected for) because those negative responses to incest would lead to a survival advantage over those individuals without such negative responses. Third, the eventual dominance of such feelings of revulsion toward incest in humans of all cultures would be incorporated into a universal moral/ethical rule against this behavior (Boyd, 2004a, p. 229). It is important to note, however, that according to this perspective, the taboo against incest did not come from outside human experience, but is a result of the Darwinian mechanisms of random variation (of genes) and natural selection.

E.O. Wilson, the person most responsible for bringing an evolutionary perspective to the study of social behaviors such as morality, suggests that the origin of ethics comes down to accepting that ethical precepts are either human inventions (what he calls the empirical approach) or that they are independent of human experience and are given from a source outside the human mind, a position he calls 'the transcendentalist perspective' (Wilson, 1998, p. 260). Being an empiricist, Wilson argues for a biological approach to the study of ethics and morality, an approach that will ultimately result in a 'wiser and more enduring ethical consensus' (p. 262) than has occurred from viewing morality as coming from a transcendent source like God. Moral and ethical behaviors do not exist, according to Wilson, because of any promised heavenly reward or because of divine command. They exist because they have survival advantage. Genes that predispose individuals toward cooperation, empathy, attachment and so on will be selected and eventually predominate in humans (p. 276). Because humans cannot survive outside of a social community, we must behave in socially acceptable ways, according to social customs, mores and ethics: 'Ethical and religious beliefs are created from the bottom up, from people to their culture. They do not come from the top down, from God or other nonmaterial source to the people by way of culture' (p. 270). (As noted in this quote, not only ethics, but religion, too, is a product of evolution, a topic we will discuss in the next section of this chapter.)

Is it possible that at least some aspects of our morality and ethical behavior evolved as EP suggests? If so, does this nullify the belief that what is right and wrong is revealed by God as traditional Christianity maintains? Do we have to choose, as Wilson insists, between viewing morality as a transcendentalist or as an empiricist? Perhaps we can, as Christians, believe that God is the source of moral principles, but that moral and ethical behavior is controlled by neural mechanisms that have evolved in ways illuminated by the speculations of evolutionary psychologists. Is not human moral behavior complex enough that each of these perspectives (and perhaps others as well) might contain some truth? As discussed in other chapters of this book, we do not necessarily have to select between one approach (for example, the perspective and theories provided by EP) and another supposedly 'contradictory' explanation such as that supplied by a theological understanding of morality. Perhaps both are true. If we humans are multileveled creatures (physical, psychological, relational, spiritual), would we not have to examine a complex system of behaviors such as morals and ethics from multiple perspectives (Looy, 2004, pp. 220-21)? Maybe the ultimate or primary explanation for morality and ethics is God's revelation of his purposes for his creatures, whereas part of the proximate or secondary explanation is provided by an evolutionary account (as well as other perspectives provided by disciplines such as sociology).

Religion

According to Wilson, religion is also a product of evolution, and developed along a similar path to morality and ethics. To understand the origin of religion, according to Wilson, we must begin by considering the instinctive and biological basis for (1) belief in a permanent existence, (2) attempts to exercise control over life, and (3) identification with a particular social group. With the evolution and increasing complexity of the brain, higher-level cognitive abilities emerge, and among those abilities is the understanding that life is temporal and will not last. We are conscious of our own mortality, yet we long for permanence, and it is because of this longing that religious beliefs about life after death have developed. Our brains have also evolved a tendency to find order in our environment. Even if there is no pattern or order, for example in a series of random numbers, we are motivated to impose an order and 'see' a pattern. This tendency reflects a biological bias toward trying to control one's environment and the events in one's life, and can also be seen as an instinctive basis for the religious belief that there is a purpose or reason for the events that occur to us. Some thing or some body is in control. We are also, as discussed Chapter 3, prepared biologically to make connections or bonds with others, and without these connections we can suffer physically, psychologically and behaviorally (Commission on Children at Risk, 2003). These connections can be exclusive, in that certain behaviors or beliefs become important in identifying members as in religious denominations. Because we are biologically prepared to seek control over events in our life, to belong or connect to particular groups, and because our minds desire permanence even though we know we are mortal beings, Wilson argues religious beliefs are universal (Wilson, 1998, p. 281). Religion is invented in all cultures and across all societies because these religious beliefs are instinctive and needed. Some have argued that if religion were purely a cultural phenomenon and not related to biology at all, then religious behaviors and beliefs would not have survived. The religious expressions would have died off long ago (Grinde, 1998).

If the basis for religious belief and behavior is biological in nature, and if the emergence of such beliefs and behaviors can be understood from an evolutionary perspective, then one might expect to see correspondence between human religious practice and certain animal behaviors. Wilson speculates, for example, that instances of animal dominance and subordination resemble human submission to civil and religious authority (Wilson, 1998, p. 283). Confident and charismatic leaders, like the alpha male in an animal pack, have followers who depend upon them and follow their guidance. Members of religious cults and sects follow their leaders, at times even unto death (for example, Jim Jones and Jonestown, Heaven's Gate, and the Branch Davidians), and this subordination and obedience reflects, according to Wilson, our primate heritage (p. 284).

Wilson's argument that our biological human nature is relevant to religion and that our genetic and evolutionary histories help to explain religious beliefs and behaviors might strike some as undermining a more traditionally accepted view of religion. Indeed, Wilson himself sees the empiricist perspective he advocates as being a clear alternative for the transcendentalist viewpoint he hopes to replace. He does concede that we cannot live without these religious beliefs because the human mind 'evolved to believe in the gods' (Wilson, 1998, p. 286) and people need a sacred story, a story of purpose provided by religious tradition. His preferred sacred narrative, however, is one provided by evolutionary theory and biology, a narrative that 'possesses more content and grandeur than all religious cosmologies combined' (p. 289).

Viewing religious faith as rooted in biology might make some Christians feel uncomfortable, in that it seems to denigrate faith and makes religious belief something that is uncontrollable and unchangeable, like some innate reflex. Christians, in Western culture at least, tend to think of the body and the spirit as two separate substances, and the things of the spirit are of greater value and are to be preferred (Looy, 2005, p. 113). Certainly, the thinking goes, religious belief is a spiritual, not a biological or physical phenomenon. The biological basis of religious beliefs and behaviors that Wilson details, however, is what one would expect if there really is a God, as historical Christianity maintains, who created human beings for the purpose of relationship. An innate or intuitive spirituality would be expected if God's purpose in creation (whatever mechanism he might have used to accomplish that creation) was to have a sentient being with whom he could establish a relationship. In addition, we are embodied creatures, and our behaviors, thoughts, feelings and so on are a product of our bodily existence as well as our environment. All of our behaviors result from a dynamic interaction of biology and environment. Even the genes themselves can be 'turned on' or 'turned off' by environmental factors, so to say that a particular behavior has a genetic or biological cause is not to say that the behavior is genetically or biologically determined. This is also true, of course, for religious thoughts, beliefs, attitudes and behaviors.

One of the basic planks of the report by the Commission on Children at Risk (2003, p. 25) is that the beginning of morality is found in attachments between the infant and its caregiver(s), and that these attachments are biologically primed. Attachments are formed between an infant (under 2 years old) and one or more adult caregivers. According to the pioneer in attachment research John Bowlby, these bonds form as a result of a biological system which functions to maintain proximity between the newborn infant and an adult who will provide its care. This attachment system includes behavioral responses (for example, crying, cooing) which bring an adult to the infant, as well as behaviors (for example, crawling) which take the infant to the caregiver. In both cases, proximity is promoted. In addition to the behavioral responses, attachments involve emotional responses such as protest when the caregiving figure leaves the infant, and anxiety in the presence of strangers. When an attachment has been formed, the caregiver becomes a 'secure base' from which the infant can feel safe to explore its environment. Instead of 'clinging' to the attachment figure, a securely attached child is more independent and free to leave the caregiver for short periods of time (for example, playing in another room), trusting that the caregiver will be available if and when needed. The caregiver is a source of security for the child.

Biology prepares the infant (and the new mother as well) to begin the process of forming these crucial bonds so that the probability of the infant's survival can be improved; the infant's survival is dependent on finding someone to take care of its physical, social and psychological needs. Not only is an infant's survival dependent on the infant finding an adult to care for it, it is out of these bonds that basic trust is formed and, ultimately, consciousness emerges. It is our biological inheritance, in part, that promotes the development of moral reasoning through these early infant–caregiver attachments. Different attachment patterns can influence the child's view of the world and how the child determines what is right and what is wrong. According to Faber (2004, pp. 91–4), these attachments eventually influence our 'religious narrative', our understanding of God's role in our lives, and our responses to life's challenges and opportunities. These religious views are closely related to our early implicit (or nonconscious) memory. Is our view of God one of a loving, heavenly, caregiving Father? If so, Faber argues, this 'core narrative' develops out of early, pre-autobiographical memories of our attachment experiences. While we do not have any conscious access to these memories, the attachment patterns are nevertheless mapped onto our implicit memories, and emerge in the form of religious narratives from which, in part, we develop our picture and understanding of God. Despite the importance of biology in attachment and the role of attachment in forming these 'religious narratives', Faber argues, rather unconvincingly, that there is no reason to think that humans are 'wired for God' or that there is any biological need for faith, suggesting instead that such statements represent 'wishful, natural misperception' of the evidence (Faber, 2004, p. 207).

Of course, there will no doubt be other factors involved (for example, the environment, the work of the Holy Spirit), but might there be an innate religiosity or spirituality? When added to other evidence (for example, the work of David Hay and Alister Hardy discussed in Chapter 6), an argument for such a 'lure of the divine' seems a reasonable conclusion, not proved, but certainly reasonable. One cannot convincingly 'prove' either position with empirical evidence. A reasonable interpretation of the evidence can lead one to the position of Faber, that while there is a biological basis for attachment and while there is a link between attachment and one's religious narrative, there is no biological basis for a need for faith. On the other hand, one can interpret the same evidence, along with the work of others such as Hay mentioned above, and conclude that such a pattern of links between religious belief and biology is what one would expect if we were 'wired for God', as some have put it. Certainly, such evidence supports a position that God made us embodied creatures and that we were made for a relationship with him. Either way, science ultimately cannot provide the answer. Science can supply evidence, but one can reasonably interpret that evidence either way. One interpretation is no more 'scientific' than the other.

Another psychologist who uses attachment theory and evolutionary psychology to try to understand religion is Lee Kirkpatrick of the College of William and Mary. Kirkpatrick sees attachment theory as valuable because it is explanatory and scientific. Attachment theory not only describes how infants and caregivers (typically mothers, but not always) develop a bond, it also offers a perspective on why humans form these important relationships. In addition, numerous empirical research studies support attachment theory and the hypotheses it generates, making it, according to Kirkpatrick, thoroughly scientific. Most important, however, is the advantage that attachment theory fits comfortably into the metanarrative provided by evolutionary psychology (Kirkpatrick, 2005, pp. 18–22).

Using attachment theory and EP, Kirkpatrick develops the viewpoint that a person's relationship with God is molded, in part, by the attachment systems that function to establish bonds between infants and adult caregivers. In what ways does Kirkpatrick see God serving as an attachment figure? First, as an infant seeks to maintain contact with the adult caregiver, a religious believer seeks to maintain proximity to God through prayer, rituals and meditation. In addition, God becomes a 'secure base' for the religious believer, providing comfort in times of illness, distress and even death (Kirkpatrick, 2005, pp. 56–65). For Kirkpatrick, these similarities between God and an attachment figure are more than superficial. This attachment with God influences our thoughts, beliefs and reasoning about God (p. 56), so understanding attachment, particularly from within an EP metanarrative, is important in understanding religion, its development and expression. It is important to emphasize here that the attachment system did not evolve in order that humans could form a relationship with God. The attachment system serves the purpose of developing relationships between infants and adult caregivers, a biologically necessary function. The system was co-opted for developing religious relationships. This is an example – one of many, according to Kirkpatrick – of religion as an evolutionary by-product of a mechanism which evolved for other, nonreligious functions (pp. 236, 336).

While Kirkpatrick sees religion as a nonadaptive by-product, evolutionary theory actually provides several hypotheses about religion, some of which see religion as nonadaptive, and some of which see religion as an evolutionary adaptation. For example, evolutionary biologist David Sloan Wilson argues in his book *Darwin's Cathedral* that religion is a group-level adaptation, meaning that the level of selection is for the group, rather than the individual. Other adaptation hypotheses of religion include selection at the level of the individual and religion as a cultural 'virus', as proposed and actively advocated by Richard Dawkins. In addition to the nonadaptive hypothesis that religion is a by-product, another nonadaptive hypothesis sees religion as being maladaptive in modern society, even though it might have been adaptive in smaller premodern societies (Wilson, 2002, p. 45). Clearly, there is no single evolutionary account of religion with which all evolutionary biologists or psychologists agree. The empirical evidence that exists is interpreted differently by various evolutionary scientists.

As is the case with EP accounts of other phenomena, the 'explanations' of religion offered by Faber (2004) and Kirkpatrick (2005), as well as others such as Boyer (2001), make interesting stories, and there is some empirical or scientific evidence that can be interpreted, as these authors do, to support their positions. The empirical evidence that exists, however, is not as great as some in the EP movement would have the readers of their articles and books believe. In addition, the same evidence used to support the EP perspective can often be interpreted in ways that are not consistent with an EP account of religion. Much of the EP literature is speculation – interesting speculation, but speculation nevertheless – based on some empirical findings. This not to say the EP story is completely wrong. We are biological creatures, and we should expect that our religion will be, in part, embodied. To this extent, Christians can read the EP theories of religion 'with a grain of salt', believing that the story it tells is not complete.

Biology of God

Underlying any evolutionary account of religion is the question of whether or not there is an innate tendency toward religion. Are we 'wired for God', as some have claimed? Is there an innate spirituality that is suppressed by society? Is there a natural lure of the divine that draws humans toward the worship of something transcendent? The evidence that addresses these questions, as one might guess, is viewed differently by different scientists. Some argue (for example, Faber) that such thinking is merely wishful thinking. Like Freud in the early twentieth century, these individuals argue that religious believers want there to be a father-like being to protect them and to serve as an attachment figure, and so use projection when they see evidence for an innate spirituality in the scientific literature. Clearly, the argument goes, there is no God, so interpreting evidence for a biological basis for belief must be false, a grand wish. Is a person justified in seeing evidence in the scientific literature for a biological basis for religion or to see spirituality as, at least in part, a natural phenomenon?

Ultimately, whether or not scientific evidence supports a biological basis for belief in God or for religion is not answerable by science. That is to say, the empirical evidence can reasonably be interpreted either for or against such a view, and neither position is more 'scientific' than the other. A person can be an honest scientist, or a person who is interested in and appreciative of empirical data, and interpret such data as supporting a physical basis for belief in God or the transcendent. One can also be a scientist, or a nonscientist respectful of empirical evidence, and interpret the same evidence as not supporting a biological belief in God or the transcendent.

Hardy's hypothesis that religious or spiritual awareness is a biological trait that evolved in humans through the process of natural selection finds greater support in the empirical literature than competing social hypotheses of religion such as Freud's view that religion is a neurosis (Hay, 1994, p. 5). As discussed in Chapter 9, the current literature suggests that religiosity and spirituality are associated with higher levels of mental (and physical) health, not, as Freud's hypothesis predicts, with poorer mental health functioning. Hay found a high percentage of the population he measured responding affirmatively to questions regarding an awareness of the presence of God, or awareness of a sacred presence in nature, or receiving help in answer to prayer, or a perception of unity or oneness. These perceptions occur in a culture (Hay primarily studies the United Kingdom) that is becoming increasingly secular and where the institutional Church is experiencing decline. Nevertheless, the percentage of respondents in the United Kingdom who reported such religious/spiritual experiences and perceptions actually increased from around 48 percent to greater than 76 percent from 1987 to 2000 (Hay and Socha, 2005, p. 590), and there is evidence that this increase in spirituality is to be found in other countries around the world as well. So while the practice of organized religion might be decreasing, the presence of spirituality and the incidence of spiritual experience seems on the upswing. Granted, spiritual experience is probably more difficult to define and conceptualize than religious experience. When attempts are made to operationalize the terms, however, the surprising prevalence of spirituality and spiritual experience is seen, despite an increasing secularization of the culture and declining attendance at religious institutions such as churches, synagogues and temples. Again, one way to interpret these data is to understand them as reflecting a natural awareness of a transcendence based on our biological makeup, perhaps including neural mechanisms utilized for this purpose (see Chapter 6).

According to Hay and Socha (2005), the evidence suggests that spiritual experience is natural and widespread, particularly in children who have 'not yet been fully socialized into secular ways of interpreting reality' (p. 596). Children, even when not raised in religious homes or exposed to religious views, nevertheless tend to demonstrate a spiritual awareness that is unlikely to come from socialization, suggesting to Hay and Socha a biological basis for such experiences. The authors argue that the methodologies of prayer, contemplation and meditation – central practices of the major spiritual traditions – include an awareness of the here and now, an awareness of mystery, and an awareness of value, and it is these traits that characterize children's views of reality. This 'relational consciousness' represents a biologically based and evolved pattern that has been selected because it functions to increase cooperation and community, resulting in ethical and moral sensitivity. In other words, spirituality is seen by Hay and Socha as a natural and biological adaptation that increases survival. Their view does not eliminate the role of social factors in the expression of spirituality; it does, however, emphasize the importance of studying spirituality (and religion) at a naturalistic level in order to obtain a more complete (and nonreductionistic) understanding of the phenomenon (p. 607).

Implications for Traditional Christian Beliefs

Some contemporary theologians have considered the implications of EP for important concepts within Christian theology. For example, how does an acceptance of EP (or even some of its ideas) affect a Christian understanding of the doctrine of original sin and the fall? What are the implications of EP and evolutionary theory on our view of the *imago Dei*? Finally, how are beliefs regarding the origin of evil affected by the ideas coming from EP?

Evolutionary theory and evolutionary psychology suggest that human behavior is a function (in large part) of selection pressures that existed 100,000 years ago. In other words, in order to get a clear understanding of why we humans act the way we do, for example do good deeds, enter into monogamous relationships, parent our (or other's) children, and even aggress against others, we must consider that these behaviors are a product of the social and physical environment that existed hundreds of millennia ago. Both our good and our bad behavior are the result of random variation in genes and natural selection. The doctrines of the fall and original sin, however, say that our original parents, Adam and Eve, were created innocent and without sin and placed in the Garden of Eden where all of their needs were met.

Despite the 'perfected' state of their existence, however, they were disobedient and sinned by eating from the tree of the knowledge of good and evil. Because of this disobedience, Adam and Eve were removed from the Garden of Eden, sin became part of our human nature and evil entered the world.

Related to the fall and original sin is the doctrine of the *imago Dei*. Humans are made in the image of God, and it is this image that makes humans unique among all of God's creation. Yes, humans are part of the natural order, and yes, humans are similar to animals in many ways, but humans are also different in important respects. We are 'like' God in that we are made in his image. Even though the phrase 'image of God' appears only three times in the Hebrew Bible (Shults, 2003, p. 219), this doctrine is a key tenet of the Christian faith, and is central to a Christian understanding of human nature. Who or what we are as human beings is a question addressed more fully in Chapter 7; however, for present purposes we need to consider what the implications of EP might be to this important Christian concept.

The doctrine of *imago Dei* emerges out of and is a part of the doctrines of the fall and original sin, and can be thought of as part of the standard Western view of human nature, a picture that not only incorporates a theory of the body in relation to the soul (a dualistic model), but also includes a view of creation based upon the first three chapters of Genesis. This Western view (largely developed by Augustine, who pulled together the work of other theologians, biblical interpretations and Church teachings) sees the earth as being created as perfect, with no natural evil or mortality. Adam and Eve, as mentioned above, were perfect in all ways and were immortal. As a result of the fall, however, physical and spiritual death entered into the world. Adam and Eve were no longer immortal (physical death), nor were they perfect (spiritual death). The guilt and depravity of this original sin is conveyed to all subsequent humans; in addition, evil entered the world and affected creation itself. So human nature is depraved, evil and totally without hope except through the unmerited grace of God.

While different in important ways from some earlier positions held by the Church, Augustine's views became part of the Western Church's accepted teachings, and heavily influenced later theologians such as John Calvin. This familiar view of human nature, however, has not gone unchallenged by some contemporary theologians and is not the only biblical view proposed. Other perspectives, it is argued, are not only supported biblically, but are more coherent with current philosophical thinking and scientific evidence (Shults, 2003, pp. 189–216; Williams, 2001, pp. 48–62), and are also consistent with and supportive of the notion of natural law as developed by Thomas Aquinas (Boyd, 2004b, p. 677).

For example, another tradition in the Christian Church, coming more from an Eastern Christian influence, sees the earth as created not perfect, but innocent. Adam and Eve were not created perfect or immortal, but were made by God as mortal children, with the potential to grow and develop in knowledge and character. Physical death did not enter into the world as a result of the fall, it was already part of the creation. What did result from the fall, however, was the spiritual death of Adam and Eve, who became separated from God and could no longer develop the kind of knowledge and character God envisioned for his human creation.

Much of Western Christianity followed the Augustinian theory of human nature; however, Eastern Orthodox (and Judaism for that matter) did not. So the 'implication of such a theory [Augustinian] from biblical texts is not automatic or necessary' (Shults, 2003, p 192). Many scholars of the Bible do not believe that humans were originally without sin, that the creation was created perfect or that the fall resulted in the introduction of mortality and death. These scholars point out that it was only after eating the forbidden fruit that Adam and Eve developed the knowledge of good and evil (Genesis 3:22); if they were created perfect, so the argument goes, they would have already known what was good and what was evil. How could perfect people not know right from wrong? Also, Adam and Eve were not created immortal, because they were sent out of the garden before they could eat of the fruit of the Tree of Life and live for ever (Genesis 3:22–23).

As mentioned above, according to the received view of the fall, evil entered the world through the disobedience of Adam and Eve forever affecting human nature, our relationships with others, our relationship to God and our relationship with the rest of creation. The existence of evil, however, remains a problem for many Christians. If God is all-knowing and all-powerful, he would have known that Adam and Eve would sin, and could have stopped them. The fact that he did not implies that God is complicit in the introduction of evil into the world, which would make God less that completely good, which is another accepted description of God's nature. Some have concluded that either God is good and evil is contrary to his plan, or God is all-powerful and evil is part of his plan and his desire for this life. If the latter is the case, then all natural evils (for example, earthquakes, hurricanes, Tsunamis, diseases) as well as all human-generated evils (for example, wars, rapes, killings) are willed by God and are part of God's plan. Yes, Adam and Eve sinned, but God could have created a world where Adam and Eve could not have sinned. He did not, so evil is ultimately from God and part of his creation.

An alternative view is that God surrenders some of his sovereignty and gives human beings freedom. God, according to this position, does not control all and does not know all. God takes risks with his relationships with humans (Sanders, 1998, pp. 9–14). So God gave Adam and Eve freedom to choose between good and evil, and did not know what their decision would be. Therefore, God was 'sorry that he had made man on the earth' when 'every imagination of the thoughts of his [man's] heart was only evil continually' (Genesis 6:5–6). This outcome was not God's intent or will, and evil is not part of God's plan or his purpose for mankind. Evil (neither natural nor human-generated) is not from God; it is a result of human decision to rebel against God.

From an evolutionary theory perspective, evil is the imposition of fitness costs on another individual or group. In other words, evil acts are those that decrease the reproductive success of another person or group (Duntley and Buss, 2004, pp. 103–4). For example, at the extreme end of a continuum of evil would be murder, because that behavior exacts the most excessive costs to reproductive success of the person killed. However, the amount of evil in such acts is modulated by the degree of relatedness (genetic, tribal, national and so on) one has to the victim or by 'extenuating' circumstances such as killing in self-defense or to save one's family (that is, protecting one's own genes). Good, on the other hand, consists of acts that result in an increase in fitness to the recipient, for example one's children, relatives or friends (Duntley and Buss, 2004, pp. 115–16).

How might one reconcile this account of evil presented by EP with a biblical perspective? One approach is to argue that as one studies nature, evolution (God's mechanism for creation) seems to result in greater and greater intelligence, variety and autonomy (Morris, 2003), resulting in the human species, which is, as far as we know, the only species with the ability to think about and reflect upon the morality of its own behavior and to adjust its behavior accordingly (Williams, 2001, pp. 163–5). We humans can also make judgments about (perhaps through the activity of mirror neurons, to be discussed in Chapter 10) the moral and ethical behavior of others. As Williams (2001) puts it: 'Morality develops naturally … With our evolution, a remarkable capacity for morality enters the universe. Like God, we know good from evil' (p. 166). The biblical story tells of Adam and Eve eating of the tree of knowledge of good and evil. EP sees that knowledge coming through an evolutionary process. Both stories of evil (and good) can be true. A Christian does not have to choose between them. Both tell of a broken relationship with God, a relationship that can only be restored through the Good News of the gospels.

Beyond Evolutionary Psychology

> Evolution, then, is the creation myth of our age. By telling us our origins it shapes our views of what we are. It influences not just our thought, but our feelings and actions too, in a way which goes far beyond its official function as a biological theory. To call it a myth does not of course mean that it is a false story. It means that is has great symbolic power, which is independent of its truth. (Midgley, 2002, p. 33)

As the quote by philosopher Mary Midgley suggests, evolution is more than a biological theory in our society, it functions as a story of origins. To some, EP serves a similar function, in that it purports to explain the origin of human behavior, including complex social behavior. One criticism of evolutionary psychology is that in its attempt to account for all behavior, EP tries to explain too much, becoming an unwieldy behavioral 'theory of everything'. Another criticism of EP and its emphasis on genetic variation and natural selection is that it suggests a biological or genetic fatalism. That is to say, some might read the literature on EP and come to the conclusion that there is nothing one can do about behavior because it is all determined by genes and biology. While some writers of EP books and articles contribute either explicitly or implicitly to this notion, this view is not a correct understanding of EP. Genes and the environment work together. The environment can contribute to turning some genes on and turning other genes off. So genetics or biology is not destiny.

EP has also been criticized because of the close connection it makes between humans and other animals. It is true that science, perhaps especially evolutionary science, has narrowed the separation between humans and animals. At the same time, however, evolutionary science has also illuminated the ways in which humans and animals are importantly and critically different. Language remains a uniquely human ability, differing not only in degree, but also in kind compared to animal communication. Many species of animals are remarkably intelligent, but as is true with language, human intelligence also differs in kind from the intelligence seen in animals. While there is some controversy on this point, it seems fairly clear that the human mind is 'radically different' and that even nonhuman primates do not have the intellectual capacity for moral reasoning, theory of mind, personal self-awareness, awareness of the transcendent, or second-order intentionality which permits the interpretation of complex social behaviors to emerge (Fisher, 2005, p. 300). It should not surprise us that we share with animals many important genetic, biological, emotional and cognitive features, because we, like the animals, are from the earth (Genesis 1 and 2). While the stories of EP are interesting and make some sense, they seem too contrived at times, and EP theorists often engage in speculation rather than analysis of hard empirical data, which are frequently lacking. Nevertheless, EP reminds us of our biological natures. Because we are of the same 'stuff' as the other animals, we should expect some commonalities between humans and animals. This is particularly true if, as much of the evidence suggests, evolution was the mechanism God used to create.

The universality of religion, according to Wilson and other proponents of evolutionary psychology, is a product of the evolved human brain and mind. Whether there are cognitive mechanisms that evolved specifically for a religious purpose or whether cognitive mechanisms evolved for other functions and were co-opted for religious purposes is a point of disagreement, and the existing evidence relevant to this question can and has been argued both ways (Kirkpatrick, 2005, pp. 214–39). Regardless of how one interprets the evidence, a spiritually inclined brain, however it might have developed, is what one would expect if God created us for the purpose of having a relationship with him. If this account is true, one would expect religious beliefs and behaviors to have adaptive advantages, and indeed, one can make the argument that religiosity and/or spirituality does provide such selective benefits. For example, religions tend to promote cooperative social relations among believers, generally healthy lifestyles and positive psychological states. In fact, there is a growing literature that religiosity/spirituality is associated with improved mental and physical health as well as increased longevity, and from the viewpoint of EP, those are certainly outcomes that carry a selective advantage. The next chapter discusses what are for some people the surprising and unexpected research findings regarding the healthful effects of religion and spirituality.

Chapter 9

Religion/Spirituality and Health

Mark suffered a heart attack two days ago and is in a coronary care unit (CCU) at a large medical center. He has access to the best medical care available in the country. His cardiologist is highly trained and has twenty years of experience, the CCU is fitted with the best technology money can buy, and the nursing staff on the unit is of the highest quality. The medical center is also a research hospital, and one of the projects in which the hospital is involved is a study on the effects of intercessory prayer on cardiac patient outcomes. The researchers want to know whether cardiac patients who are unknowingly prayed for will have shorter CCU stays and fewer complications than patients for whom intercessory prayer is not offered.

Mark is randomly assigned to the prayer group in which four 'intercessors' pray, over the next thirty days, for Mark's uncomplicated recovery. Other CCU patients are randomly assigned to either the prayer or the no prayer conditions. During the next month, Mark's physical status, along with the other patients in the prayer group, is assessed and compared to that of the no prayer control group. The study follows what is called a blinded procedure, in that no one – not Mark, his doctors or even the researchers themselves – knows whether Mark is in the prayer or no prayer condition. The intercessors do not know Mark, and have no contact with him; they simply have agreed to pray for his speedy recovery.

Some studies like this one suggest that prayer is associated with better medical outcomes (Byrd, 1988; Harris et al., 1999). The differences in outcome between the prayer and no prayer groups are typically small, but they do reach what scientists call statistical significance, meaning that the differences are most likely not due to chance. In other words, there seems to be a 'real' effect of prayer. Other research, however, shows no effect of intercessory prayer on recovery from physical illness. A recent study by Benson et al. (2006) compared three groups of patients who were recovering from coronary artery bypass graft surgery. One group received intercessory prayer after being told that they might or might not receive prayer, one group did not receive prayer after being told that they might or might not be prayed for, and a third group received prayer after being told that they would be prayed for by others. The first two groups of patients (the prayer and no prayer groups) did not differ in the number of complications they experienced after the surgery (which is what the experimenters were measuring). The third group, however, the group that knew they were being prayed for, experienced more complications than the groups which were uncertain about receiving intercessory prayer (Benson et al., 2006, p. 934).

Studies such as these are often criticized on a couple of fronts. First, from a researcher's standpoint, how can one be sure that those patients in the no prayer group are, in fact, not being prayed for? Although the intercessors in the study are not praying for those patients, perhaps friends and family members of the patients are. Second, from a theological standpoint, do we really think that God is either going to intervene or not intervene based upon whether a person is in the experimental or the control group of a research study? Can we get control of God in such a fashion?

While these kinds of research projects have been criticized, others have praised them as examples of how one might go about determining the extent to which there is a relationship between religion and health (both mental and physical). As we will see below, interest in this subject has grown over the past decade, and the outcome of this kind of research offers some surprising results. Not only is the effect of religion on health a hot topic of research in psychology, neuroscience, medicine and related fields (the United States government has spent over $2 million on so-called 'distant healing' effects over the past five years), so too is research into forgiveness and its effect on health. Just what is forgiveness, what effect does it have on one's health and well-being, and how can the offer of forgiveness and its acceptance be encouraged? These are questions researchers are now investigating, in part because money is now available to support these studies, and the money is available because there are public health reasons for understanding how mental and physical health can be improved and for encouraging forgiveness, both on the interpersonal as well as on a larger social or cultural scale.

This chapter will first review some of the literature on the relationship between religion or spirituality and health. In the past, largely due to the influence of a Freudian view of religion within psychology and psychiatry, religion was assumed to have a negative influence on mental health, and probably physical health as well. Belief in God was an illusion that, like other false beliefs, needed to be corrected. Freud believed that it was unhealthy to have these illusions, and that they would eventually cause psychological problems. The findings of much of the religion and health literature suggest just the opposite: that religion and spirituality are, in fact, correlated with positive mental and physical health outcomes.

After a review of this literature, we will then look at the subject of forgiveness, a topic of fundamental importance in Christianity, Judaism and other world religions. Like the research on religion and health, a substantial literature on forgiveness has developed over the past decade or so. Some researchers are interested in how many different types of forgiveness exist, others in how forgiveness can be encouraged. Still others are investigating the physiological effects of forgiveness, and how any positive effects of forgiveness on the body might be mediated. These two general areas of research are relatively new to psychology and neuroscience, and they illustrate how issues of importance to religion are now being studied in both the human and natural sciences. While once, not so very long ago, these topics were considered taboo for a scientist, subjects such as these are now fair game for science to study. The encouragement to investigate these topics is provided, in many cases, by money supplied by either private or governmental sources.

Religion and Spirituality Defined in the Literature

In the literature discussed in this chapter, researchers typically look at the relationships between mental and/or physical health and religion and spirituality. The terms 'religion' and 'spirituality' therefore need to be defined, and several attempts to do so have been made, with varying success. Both religion and spirituality are multifaceted, and neither is easily conceptualized. Koenig, McCullough and Larson in their authoritative handbook define and distinguish religion and spirituality by conceptualizing religion as 'an organized system of beliefs, practices, rituals, and symbols' designed to increase one's closeness to something considered to be sacred or transcendent and to facilitate a greater awareness of how one is interconnected with and responsible to others living in the same community. Spirituality is conceptualized as a personal quest for meaning and greater understanding about life and relationships to the transcendent which may or may not result in religious practices. Religion, therefore, is considered to be community-focused, formal and organized, oriented toward behavior and practice, institutional and doctrinal. Spirituality, on the other hand, is more individualistic, emotional and subjective, and less systematic, organized, authoritarian and doctrinal (Koenig, McCullough and Larson, 2001, p. 18).

However, making these kinds of distinctions between religion and spirituality can be problematic, in that there is the sense among some that spirituality is 'good' while religion is 'bad', a division that at best is overly simplistic. In addition, there is overlap between religion and spirituality that is lost in such a clear-cut differentiation. For example, while religion might be more institutional and community-focused than spirituality typically is, it is nevertheless the case that both take place in a social context that affects the practice of one's religion or spirituality. Also, while spirituality might be more subjective and personal, religion also contains elements of individuality and subjectivism. Finally, for most people, spirituality is experienced within a religious context, and a clear distinction between the two is simply not perceived (Hill and Pargament, 2003, p. 64). Religion and spirituality are related for most people; they are not polar opposites as is sometimes suggested or inferred by attempts to measure these concepts.

While some researchers attempt to assess religiosity by measuring churchgoing behavior or frequency of prayer and scripture reading, most recognize that any valid and reliable measure of religion and/or spirituality must consider the multifaceted nature of these concepts. A recent review of 125 measures of religion and spirituality (Hill and Hood, 1999) shows the tremendous breadth of the terms as well as the great variety of the measurement approaches taken by researchers over the years. The review includes measurements of religion and spirituality that assess beliefs, attitudes, religious development and orientation, coping mechanisms, mysticism and views of life after death, to mention just a few. These are paper-and-pencil measures where a person fills out a questionnaire which is later scored by a researcher. While the scoring system varies depending on the specific questionnaire, typically the higher the score on the specific measure, the higher the religiosity or spirituality of the participant. These religiosity and spirituality scores are then correlated with other measures of the subject's mental or physical health.

As is true of any self-report measure, the pencil-and-paper questionnaires used in the study of religion and health are subject to methodological problems, including limitations of comprehension, memory errors and social desirability. For example, a person completing a questionnaire on religiosity might not understand adequately what is meant by some of the terms on the survey. Reading levels vary, sometimes dramatically, from person to person, which makes constructing a questionnaire that can be used for a wide range of subjects difficult. In addition, a person may not remember with enough detail to correctly answer a particular question. Finally, social desirability refers to the tendency for participants filling out a questionnaire to respond to a particular question in a manner that makes them appear in a desirable light, for example saying they go to church an average of once per week when, in fact, church attendance is more accurately once per month. As a result of these limitations inherent in self-report procedures, other ways to assess religiosity are being developed, including the observing of response times as a measure of attitude accessibility (Hill and Pargament, 2003, p. 70).

Role of Religion and Spirituality in Physical Health

Recent research has investigated the role religion (and/or spirituality) has in physical health. In order to answer this question definitively, one must conduct a true experiment where there is random assignment of subjects to conditions (for example, religious/nonreligious), manipulation of an independent variable (for example, introduce the religious variable to those subjects in the 'religious' group and withhold it from subjects in the 'nonreligious' group) and control of all known other variables that might influence the outcome of the study (for example, general health of the subjects in the study). Because of the nature of the subject matter (religion and health), these randomized controlled experiments are typically not done. Instead, measures of religiosity and health are taken, and a correlation or association is made on the two measures. For example, a test is conducted to see if those subjects who score high on a particular measure of religiosity also score high on a measure of overall physical health. While a causal connection cannot be made between the two variables (for example, religion and health) using this procedure, important information can be obtained.

Studies of this sort have been conducted to see if there is any relationship between religion and heart disease, cerebrovascular disease, immune system function, cancer, pain and mortality, to mention just a few of the health indices assessed. It is safe to say that mixed results are typically found, some studies showing a positive relationship between religion and physical health (that is, those who score high on religiosity have good health), some showing a negative relationship (that is, those scoring high on religiosity having poor health) and some studies showing no relationship at all between the two variables. Nevertheless, reviews of this literature are suggestive of an overall helpful effect of religion on physical health (Koenig, 1997; Koenig, McCullough and Larson, 2001; Seybold and Hill, 2001; Thoresen, 1999; Thoresen, Harris and Oman, 2001). Some of the findings include higher levels of religiosity correlated with lower rates of heart disease, cirrhosis, myocardial infarction, stroke, kidney failure, cancer mortality and overall mortality. In addition, higher religiosity is associated with lower blood pressure (both systolic and diastolic) as well as lower levels of cholesterol and chronic pain. To be sure, not all studies show these relationships, and religion can have negative effects on health, as when religious groups oppose medical care or intervention, for example the refusal to accept a transfusion that might save one's life (Lee and Newberg, 2005). The overall impression from the literature, however, is of a salutary or beneficial effect of religion (or spirituality) on physical health. Possible mechanisms for these positive effects on health will be discussed later in this chapter.

Role of Religion/Spirituality in Mental Health

While the apparent positive impact of religion on physical health might not be surprising, the historical view of the relationship between religion and mental health suggests that there should be a negative effect of religion. This view comes mainly from Sigmund Freud's opinion of religion as being a neurosis. To Freud, belief in God is an illusion based upon our wish that such a being exists (Gay, 1989, pp. 685–722). We wish there was an all-powerful and all-knowing father figure who could take care of us and protect us. We wish that good was rewarded and evil punished. We wish that there was more to existence than three score and ten years on this earth. We wish there was an afterlife in which we will live in a new Eden with God. We wish there was purpose and meaning in life. Unfortunately, according to Freud, none of these wishes is true. There is no afterlife, no meaning or purpose; evil is not always punished and good rewarded. There is no father in the sky to protect us. These are all examples of illusions that need to be eliminated from our thinking and beliefs. We need to recognize, Freud states, that it is only science that can provide knowledge. So-called revealed knowledge is false, and the sooner we recognize that fact, the better off we will be psychologically, emotionally, socially and so on. Others have also suggested that psychological problems are associated with, perhaps even caused by, religious belief and practice. According to these views, religious individuals will be more likely to experience depression, low self-esteem and other psychological problems than are nonreligious people (Watters, 1992).

The empirical literature, however, suggests that, as with physical health, mental health is also better in more religious and spiritual individuals (Gartner, Larson and Allen, 1991; Koenig, 1997; Koenig, McCullough and Larson, 2001; Levin and Chatters, 1998; Seybold and Hill, 2001). Positive associations have been found between religion/spirituality and well-being, marital satisfaction, meaning and purpose, optimism, self-esteem, and general psychological functioning. Negative associations have been found between religion/spirituality and suicide, drug and alcohol abuse, criminality, depression, anxiety and loneliness. To be sure, associations between religion and some forms of psychopathology (for example, authoritarianism, dogmatism, suggestibility and dependence) have also been found in some studies. The overall message, however, is of a positive influence of religion on mental health, a finding at odds with the 'commonsense' position held in much of psychology during the twentieth century.

Mechanisms

A number of mechanisms have been proposed to explain how religious belief might have a positive effect on physical and mental health. One way in which religiosity might affect health is via social networks and social support. Social networks are the interrelationships among one's friends, family and associates, and much evidence suggests that the richer and fuller one's social network is, the more social support that network provides, and social support is essential to well-being. While the number of people in one's social network is important, the nature of the social relationships (positive and supportive) is equally crucial (Krantz and McCeney, 2002).

While there are many ways of receiving social support that do not involve religion, it is certainly the case that religious and spiritual communities provide opportunities for interaction and fellowship with others, and religiously involved people report receiving greater social support than the religiously uninvolved (Koenig, 2002, p. 15). Whether through formal social programs (for example, visiting the sick, feeding the hungry, building houses for the homeless), more informal activities (for example, baking cookies, chaperoning a dance for teenagers) or through weekly worship services, people actively involved in a Church community or family can provide social support to others and receive social support themselves. The recent report from the Commission on Children at Risk emphasizes the importance of making connections to other people and to moral and spiritual meaning in the overall health and development of children (Commission on Children at Risk, 2003, p. 14). These connections are important to adolescents and adults as well, and are made available in a faith community.

Lifestyle is also a mechanism through which religion and spirituality can affect physical and mental health. Religious commitment can motivate a person to adopt healthier behaviors such as abstinence from smoking, drug use and risky sexual behavior, and religious groups that do adopt a stricter behavioral lifestyle (for example, Mormons, Old Order Amish, Orthodox Jews) report a more positive health status than the population as a whole (Hill and Butter, 1995). In the case of cardiovascular disease, the greater the religiosity of the person, the lower the risk of mortality associated with the disease, and this association is mediated through the healthier lifestyle encouraged by the religious beliefs (Powell, Shahabi and Thoresen, 2003).

Psychological factors can also mediate the relationship between religion and mental and physical health. For example, variations between individuals in how they perceive a particular situation can affect later health. Those who have what Martin Seligman calls an optimistic explanatory style (perceiving negative events as externally caused and situation-specific, and positive events as internally caused and typical) tend to be more healthy than those with a pessimistic explanatory style (seeing negative events as internally caused and typical and positive events as externally caused and situation specific). Indeed, more religiously conservative people tend to be more optimistic and hopeful than more moderately religious ones, and more moderately religious people tend to be more optimistic and hopeful than the those who hold liberal religious beliefs (Sethi and Seligman, 1993). The findings regarding explanatory style and health are consistent with the evidence mentioned above that the more conservative religious practitioner (as defined by lifestyle) also tends to have a more positive health status. In addition to explanatory style, other coping strategies such as attributions of purpose and meaning to negative events, locus of control beliefs, altruistic behavior toward others in need, and acceptance from other people or from God have also been proposed as psychological factors mediating the link between religiosity and health (Koenig, McCullough and Larson, 2001; Pargament, 1997).

Some investigators suggest that physiological factors play a role in the link between religiosity and health. Negative emotional states (for example, anger and fear) activate the hypothalamic-pituitary-adrenal axis (HPA) and the sympathetic nervous system, which are involved in the stress response. Activation of these mechanisms triggers the release of stress hormones such as cortisol as well as the release of the neurotransmitter norepinephrine. Continued activation of these systems can produce physical problems (such as hypertension) and can compromise the immune system, which increases a person's susceptibility to diseases and inflammation, including Alzheimer's disease, Type 2 diabetes, cardiovascular disease, certain cancers, and conditions associated with aging (Kiecolt-Glaser et al., 2002). Positive emotions (such as forgiveness, hope, love, contentment) can promote the kinds of perceptions mentioned above (for example, optimistic explanatory style) that are linked to good health (Salovey et al., 2000), and meditation, forgiveness and some religious and spiritual thoughts and beliefs produce beneficial physiological effects (Seeman, Dubin and Seeman, 2003; Thoresen, 1999).

Social support influences health by way of a variety of physiological mechanisms, for example the cardiovascular and immune systems (Uchino, Uno and Holt-Lunstad, 1999). Stress appraisal, positive mood, health behaviors and self-esteem can modulate physiological systems, producing more positive health. Empirical research suggests that religion can serve as a coping mechanism that works via social resources, psychological processes and their mediating physiological mechanisms to produce better health in the more religious individual. While not all religious individuals are healthier than their nonreligious counterparts, and while not all religious practices are correlated with better health, the overall message of the many studies that have looked at the relationship between religion and heath (mental and physical) suggests a salutary effect.

Forgiveness

Forgiveness plays a major role in the Judeo-Christian tradition. In the Old Testament, an entire Levitical priesthood existed that performed the necessary sacrificial rituals and duties to effect the forgiveness of sins for the people of Israel. In the New Testament, Jesus Christ is described as a new kind of priest, one whose self-sacrifice once and for all secures an eternal redemption for those who believe (Hebrews 9:12). One Bible concordance consulted had over 145 references to forgiveness or related words. In the 1990s, a surge in interest in the psychology of forgiveness was seen, in large measure driven by the availability of funds from the John Templeton Foundation. Research in forgiveness was also driven by the emergence of a new area of psychology known as positive psychology, which is interested in the scientific study of optimal human functioning, virtues, health and well-being rather than the more negative aspects of human behavior and health too often characteristic of psychological research.

In the literature, forgiveness and unforgiveness are typically defined as opposing responses centering on emotions. Unforgiveness is an emotional complex characterized by bitterness, resentment, hostility, anger, fear and hatred. These unpleasant, negative emotions are thought to motivate a person to reduce unforgiveness. According to this account, unforgiveness can occur as a result of a person thinking and ruminating about a wrong that was done to them (Worthington, 2001, pp. 162–3). Forgiveness, on the other hand, is a replacement of the cold, hard emotions of unforgiveness with positive emotions such as empathy, compassion, love, humility and gratitude. According to Everett Worthington, a leading researcher in forgiveness, these positive emotions are more than mere feelings. They also involve thoughts, memories, brain activation, hormone release and muscular movement (Worthington, 2001, pp. 163–5). Replacing unforgiveness with forgiveness is a kind of reconditioning process. One cannot be angry, bitter, hostile, compassionate, loving and empathic at the same time. The cold, negative emotions of unforgiveness need to be replaced by the positive emotions (and thoughts, memories, brain activity and so on) of forgiveness. Unforgiveness can be reduced at a societal level through retaliation, revenge, personal restitution, public confession and conflict resolution, and at an intrapersonal level through denial, reframing, justifying and forgetting. True forgiveness, however, involves replacing the emotions of unforgiveness with the emotions of forgiveness, and Worthington has developed a method called REACH designed to encourage and accomplish this reconditioning process.

REACH is a five-step model to promote forgiveness, and stands for Recall, Empathy, Altruism, Commitment and Holding onto the forgiveness (Worthington, 1998, pp. 107–37). The first step in the REACH model is to *Recall the hurt*. When we remember an event in which some one has (we believe) wronged us in some way, there is an emotional response to the memory. Hormones such as cortisol are released, the brain secretes various neurotransmitters, and there may be motor responses such as muscular tension. Recalling the hurt involves remembering the hurtful event, but within a supportive environment, one where additional pain from the memory will not develop. If one can come to remember the hurt within an atmosphere of support and empathy from others, then hopefully the old emotions associated with the event (anger, bitterness and so on) will be extinguished. Such extinction is the beginning of forgiveness.

Empathizing with the person who hurt you is the second step in the REACH model. By trying to 'get into the shoes' of the person who harmed you, one can attempt to understand what they might have been thinking and feeling at the time of the hurtful event. Empathy also helps the person who was wronged come to realize that they too have done wrong to others. No one can say that they have never hurt another person's feelings or harmed another person in some way. By seeking and achieving empathy for the other, we can hopefully realize that we have needed forgiveness from others in the past and should perhaps now consider forgiveness for the person who wronged us.

Step three is to offer the *Altruistic* gift of forgiveness. By recalling how we have done wrong to others in the past and received forgiveness for that wrong, we can feel humility about ourselves and gratitude that we have received forgiveness. The REACH model sees this as a motivator toward granting forgiveness to the person who has harmed us. Offering forgiveness at this point is perhaps an altruistic gift, but it is still private. One can always deny at a later time that the gift was ever made. Step four, however, asks the person to make a public *Commitment* of this forgiveness, for example by writing a letter of forgiveness and reading the letter out loud to a supportive group. Perhaps in this public setting the person will be asked to consider the wisdom of actually sending the letter, or a version thereof, to the offender.

The last step in the REACH model is the *Holding onto forgiveness*. New physiological responses, thoughts and attitudes have hopefully been conditioned to the harmful event. Unforgiveness has been replaced by forgiveness through the various exercises included in the REACH model. It is important to understand that forgiveness, which is motivational and emotional, will not necessarily lead to reconciliation of a broken relationship. There can be reconciliation without forgiveness, and forgiveness without reconciliation. Forgiveness does, however, facilitate reconciliation, making it easier for the interpersonal relationship to be healed.

Neuropsychological Dimensions of Forgiveness

The brain impacts all behavior (motor, affective, cognitive and so on), so it is of interest to try to understand how the brain is involved in the behaviors of asking for and granting forgiveness. In order for interpersonal forgiveness to take place, several conditions must be present. First, some wrong (or perceived wrong) must be committed. When this act occurs, it is perceived as 'wrong' because someone's sense of self has been injured. If no sense of self is present, no injury to the self can occur. A threatened sense of self or self-esteem elicits anger, and is seen as a potential cause of violence, aggression and, perhaps, revenge-seeking (Baumeister, Smart and Boden, 1996). Therefore, a prerequisite for forgiveness is the injury, perceived or actual, to one's sense of self. Second, a causal link must be made between the act and the feeling of injury. In other words, the injured person must associate the act committed by another with the injured sense of self. The third condition is an emotional reaction on the part of the injured person. The injurious act must produce negative affect in the individual; the injury must feel bad to the wronged person. A final condition for interpersonal forgiveness is memory of the event. Without memory of the injury, there is no need for interpersonal forgiveness.

What brain areas are involved in producing the sense of self, causality, emotion and memory? The neural mechanisms behind the self constitute one of the great mysteries in psychology and the neurosciences (see Chapter 7). It is unlikely, however, that a single brain structure generates this sense of self. Interactions among several brain regions seamlessly produce the self. While empirical evidence is difficult to gather, some preliminary data suggest that the superior and inferior parietal lobes as well as the prefrontal cortex are areas that help to generate this sense of being a separate self (Damasio, 1999; Newberg and d'Aquili, 2001; Newberg et al., 2000).

The brain's ability to see patterns and generate causal hypotheses is due to what is called an interpreter, located in the brain's left hemisphere (Wolford, Miller and Gazzaniga, 2000). It provides causes to actions, and provides patterns to incoming stimuli. The brain evolved in an environment where finding pattern in and determining causes of events yielded survival advantages, and this tendency to see patterns and causes is so strong that it can occur even if no pattern is actually present.

Emotion is generated by a variety of brain structures located in the limbic system. A major structure responsible for emotion is the amygdala, but it works in conjunction with a number of other limbic areas such as the hypothalamus and hippocampus. Emotion is involved in the interpretation of events and the assignment of causality discussed above. If we determine that someone has wronged us and injured our sense of self, that appraisal will likely be associated with negative emotions. Whether the negative affect comes before or after the appraisal is debatable, and is at the center of theoretical differences; that the emotional response and the appraisal occur together is clear (Lazarus, 1991).

The hippocampus is also involved in the final condition for forgiveness: memory. Without the hippocampus, new declarative memories are not formed. Declarative memory consists of information we can declare or tell to others. Part of this information includes autobiographical or episodic memory, knowledge of events that have happened to us. These memories help to create the self as a long-term concept. A person who cannot remember an act that injured his sense of self feels no need for revenge. Forgiveness requires that the offender and the event are remembered.

What is the adaptive function of forgiveness? Why should we seek or grant forgiveness? Newberg and colleagues (2000) propose that the perception of a wrong committed against oneself often leads to an attempt to redress that wrong and to restore equilibrium in the relationship. The redress, however, can be viewed as excessive by the original actor, which results in further disequilibrium. Such an unchecked system can produce social chaos. Perhaps one function of forgiveness is to reduce the likelihood that hostilities between aggrieved parties will escalate. Given the findings suggesting a link between threatened self-esteem and violence (Baumeister, Smart and Boden, 1996), de-escalating revenge behavior may literally save one's life. Granting forgiveness can also generate empathy and positive feelings for the victim from outside observers (Newberg et al., 2000), increasing the individual's social status.

An additional function of forgiveness might be its association with health (Worthington, Berry and Parrott, 2001, pp. 113–21). As suggested above, there is a connection between health and social support (Uchino, Uno and Holt-Lunstad, 1999). Perhaps a person who is forgiving benefits not only from enhanced social status, but also from increased size and strength of the social network. This network, in turn, serves to buffer the stress the individual experiences and protects overall health.

Research typically investigates the involvement of psychological processes (for example, personality, development, emotion, interpersonal relationships and so on) in forgiveness. The effect of forgiveness on physical health and the disease process, however, remains unexamined, and theoretical models describing the connection between forgiveness and physical health have yet to be developed (Seybold et al., 2001; Thoresen, Harris and Luskin, 2000). The suggestion that forgiveness affects health comes, in part, from evidence that religion and spirituality play a role in both physical and mental health as discussed above.

A recent study by Witvliet, Ludwig and Vander Laan (2001) addressed the relative lack of information on forgiveness and health by studying the physiological changes that occur when people respond, using imagery, in forgiving or unforgiving ways. Unforgiving imagery (for example, rehearsing the hurt, harboring a grudge) increased the sympathetic nervous system arousal and cardiovascular reactivity characteristic of negative emotional reactions. Subjects in the unforgiving condition also showed greater amounts of anger and sadness, emotions that are risk factors for heart disease (Allen and Scheidt, 1996). Witvliet, Ludwig and Vander Laan (2001) suggest that forgiveness reduces health risks by decreasing the physiological demands associated with anger as well as hostility, a robust risk factor for coronary heart disease (Miller et al., 1996).

With an aging population in most of the industrialized world, greater demands are placed on a nation's health delivery and social welfare programs. As a result, researchers in psychology, medicine, public policy and other disciplines are interested in finding ways to improve the health of a country's population in order to reduce the stress on existing social programs. The findings reported in this chapter suggest that religion and spirituality can have a salutary effect on mental as well as physical health. To what extent religion and spirituality *per se* has a positive effect on health or whether they have their influence via psychosocial factors such as social ties and personality remains to be determined. Nevertheless these findings, along with the evidence for the innateness of spirituality discussed in Chapter 6, suggest that religion might serve an adaptive function. Understanding behavior and mental processes from an evolutionary perspective is a growing field within psychological science, as we saw in the previous chapter. It also seems to be a viewpoint that will increasingly influence our understanding of psychology and neuroscience in the future, and it is to the future of psychology, neuroscience and issues related to religion that we now turn.

Chapter 10

The Future?

> I was born human. But this was an accident of fate – a condition merely of time and place. I believe it's something we have the power to change. (Kevin Warwick, *Wired Magazine*, February 2000)

Science has made many discoveries in the past fifteen years that impact how we see ourselves as individual human beings. Some of these discoveries, as we have noted in the preceding chapters, have implications for traditional religious beliefs and practices. We have looked at the role the brain plays in religious experience and in the creation of our self or soul; we have considered the possibility that our religious beliefs emerge, at least in part, from our biology as shaped through natural selection, and we have seen how contemporary psychology and neuroscience are studying the effects of religion, spirituality and forgiveness on health. We have examined these scientific findings from the perspective that none of them present a serious challenge to religious faith. The Christian believer can openly accept confirmed scientific findings without fear that the empirical research will obviate a nonscientific or religious point of view. Reality is multilayered, and multiple perspectives are needed for a complete picture of that reality. Science provides one perspective; religious worldviews can provide others.

What about the future? Can we be as confident about what science might tell us or discover in the future? This chapter looks into the future to see what might be waiting for us over the horizon. Sometimes this future orientation will be relative short, perhaps one to five years away. Other examples we will discuss will be farther out, maybe ten to thirty years from now. Some of the material is based largely on speculation and might never occur; other examples covered, we are almost certain to see. Most of the future developments derived from research in neuroscience and psychology will not have much, if any, impact on religious beliefs and faith. Who will not rejoice if prosthetic arms can be linked to the human brain in such a way that, just like with natural limbs, merely thinking about moving the artificial arms causes their movement? Who could object if the same technology is used to help victims of amyotrophic lateral sclerosis (ALS, or Lou Gehrig's disease) move and communicate with their families? There are other developments, however, coming from psychology and cognitive science that might cause more caution, not only from Christians, but among nonbelievers as well. One such development comes from the interface of psychology, philosophy, computer science, neuroscience and other disciplines. It is a movement which seeks the evolution of the human species through a merging of the biological and the machine. We will begin this final chapter with a discussion of this challenging (and for many, troubling) movement known as transhumanism.

Transhumanism

Transhumanism can be defined as the philosophical view that human beings can and should attempt to reconfigure and remake what it means to be human. Using technology, humans should strive to self-evolve into a new kind of species, one in which biology and machine are blended. Humans will merge with their technology to become posthuman.[1]

One of the motivating principles underlying this movement is the transhumanist's belief that the carbon-based biological body is limited by the fact that it ages, becomes less and less efficient, and eventually dies. Not only the physical capabilities, but the intellectual and cognitive abilities of humans also decline with time. These deteriorations that occur with age, and even death itself, are to be avoided, and the best way to avoid them is to become a new kind of person with a new and improved body. While the early stages of this evolution from human to posthuman will involve modifying and enhancing our existing biological bodies, for example through gene modification to increase the lifespan and cognitive-enhancing drugs to improve memory, eventually a totally new kind of body will be required, a body that will not age or die. This new kind of body will be achieved through the merging of our biological body with machines until we have created the next stage in human evolution, a cyborg or robot which has the 'essentials' of human nature (love, anger, joy, fear, rationality, consciousness, spirituality), except in a 'superhuman' form. Eventually, according to these transhumanist visionaries, because a person's self or identity is essentially information in nature, we will be able to 'upload' individual personalities into these cyborgs, creating a posthuman who will enjoy immortality in a new bodily form that will never die.

Is this the stuff of science fiction? The promoters of this new vision argue that these developments will occur within the next thirty or so years. Given the increasing processing power of computers and given the greater knowledge of personhood and mind coming from contemporary research in neuroscience and psychology (see Chapter 7), these advocates of the posthuman maintain that the computers of the future will be able to process the 'information' that composes the human person, making the biological body which currently houses that information unnecessary. As Waters (2006, p. 41) puts it in his critique of the movement: 'To become posthuman requires the ability to remove the information constituting a personality from the body and to place it in a superior substratum.' That ability, the transhumanists tell us, will be realized in the lifetime of today's college student (Kurzweil, 2005, pp. 198–202).

Some might respond by saying that such a future is not possible. It is important to note, however, that we already have examples of the merging of human and technology. It is not unusual for a person to be 'enhanced' through technology in the form of eyeglasses, hearing aids or cochlear implants. Parents pay large sums

1 Examples of transhumanist and posthumanist writing can be found in Moravec (1988, 1999) and Kurzweil (2000, 2005). See also the website for the World Transhumanist Association, <http://www.transhumanism.org>. For an excellent and thoughtful critique of posthumanism from a Christian theological perspective, see Waters (2006).

of money to 'enhance' their children's memory and thinking via special courses designed to improve SAT scores. How big a step, the transhumanists ask, is it to suppose that these same parents would be willing to give their children an even greater advantage over the competition by administering drugs to increase cognitive performance or to agree to some form of genetic engineering to make their children faster and stronger on the athletic field? The current controversy over steroids in sports pales compared with what might be commonplace in ten years' time.

The ultimate posthuman vision of humanity's future portrayed by transhumanism may or may not be feasible. Despite the certainty that transhumanist writers convey about what can and will be done in the future, particularly in regards to the uploading of the human mind into a 'superior substratum', there is a great deal of doubt among neuroscientists about whether it is possible for a person's identity to exist outside the carbon-based substratum in which it is currently housed. Transhumanists maintain that the 'platform' for identity does not matter. While personhood is now embodied in a carbon-based brain, it should be possible, they argue, to store the information that makes up our mind and put that information onto a different, silicon-based platform such as a computer. As we saw in Chapter 7, however, mind and personhood seem to be intimately tied to the brain, and it is anything but clear that the mind, even if it is composed of information in the form of electrical impulses, can exist outside its biological embodiment. It just might be the case that the platform does matter.

There are points of contact between a Christian and a transhumanist worldview (for example, both see the need for human transformation, both value human life, both have a vision of eternity) in which a dialogue can develop (Campbell and Walker, 2005). Nevertheless, there are definite and important differences between how Christians view transformation, human nature, the role of the body, and eternity and how transhumanists view these subjects. For Christians, the human body is good, and is a vital part of who we are. For transhumanists, the body is a necessary (for now) evil, a view consistent with the ancient Gnostic heresy which saw the mind as imprisoned within the body, waiting to be liberated (Krueger, 2005, p. 83). Today's transhumanists are a new version of that old philosophy that was rejected by the early Church. Unlike transhumanists, Christians do not fear mortality and death, because our hope is eternal life with Christ. Eternity, according to traditional Christian belief, involves, in some admittedly mystical fashion, a resurrected body. Death is an enemy, but it is an enemy that is conquered. Our ultimate or eschatological destiny is in Christ (Waters, 2006, p. 134). For the transhumanist, it is immortality, not this notion of eternity, that is desired. Finally, the Christian sees transformation coming through Jesus Christ; for the transhumanist, self-transformation into a posthuman form is the goal.

Neuroethics

The term 'neuroethics' was coined by William Safire, former columnist for the *New York Times* and currently chairman of the Dana Foundation, a private philanthropic institute interested in brain science and in disseminating information about the personal and public benefits of brain research. The term refers to the ethical issues raised by some of the findings coming from brain research. For example, recent research on brain structure and function suggests that part of the frontal lobe, the prefrontal cortex, does not fully mature in humans until late adolescence or even early adulthood. This part of the brain is involved in making judgments, controlling impulses, and learning about the connection between behavior and outcome. If the prefrontal cortex is not fully functioning in a 15-year-old male who has committed a terrible crime, such as murder, should that young man be tried as an adult? He certainly has committed an adult crime, but what if the part of his brain that enables him to control his impulses and make appropriate judgments is not functioning at an adult level? Can or should he be held legally (or morally) responsible for his actions? Or, to take another related example, how responsible is a psychopath (a person who harms others but shows no remorse for their actions, who demonstrates no anxiety in the face of threatening conditions, or who can fake emotions to manipulate others, but who does not seem to experience genuine emotions of their own) for their illegal behavior if, as some recent research (Anderson et al., 1999; Arehart-Treichel, 2005) suggests, their prefrontal cortex is damaged or dysfunctional? To what extent is a person responsible for their behavior if the behavior is the result of a damaged brain?

Tremendous advances have been made in the ability of scientists to see inside the active brain. As discussed in Chapter 1, neuroscientists use PET, fMRI and SPECT technology to get a picture of the brain while it is performing some mental task. One of the areas in which this kind of technology is put to use is in trying to develop a new kind of 'lie detector'. What does brain activity look like when a person is telling the truth, and how is it different when that same person is lying? Will it be possible in the not-so-distant future for the police or security at the airport to determine whether a suspect or a person wanting to get on a plane is telling the truth? How about an employer using that same technology to determine whether a potential employee is 'suitable' for hire? Because we are social creatures, each of us develops a theory of what others might be thinking or feeling. Theory of Mind is important in relating to others in our social group, and there seem to be specialized cells called mirror neurons that are involved in forming this theory and developing a kind of bridge or link between minds, a link that is disrupted in individuals with autism, a disorder characterized by impairments in social interaction (Williams et al., 2001). (Mirror neurons are a class of neurons found in monkeys and in humans that fire when the monkey – or human – performs a particular behavior or sees that behavior performed by another individual (Rizzolatti and Craighero, 2004). These neurons are implicated in imitation, communication and contagious behavior as well as in developing a theory of what others are thinking, feeling or about to do.)

While our theories of what another person is thinking or feeling or what that person might do are usually pretty accurate, they are nevertheless merely good guesses. If the predictions of some neuroscientists come true, we will have even greater certainty than we do now about the content of another's thoughts and beliefs. As one commentator on neuroethics put it: 'Neuroscience holds out the latest hope of knowing what someone really thinks or feels, or what their mental condition "really" is. New technologies, particularly imaging technologies, can show us patterns of activity in the brain itself that may well prove to correlate strongly with states of mind, emotion, or thought' (Greely, 2006, p. 249). What will come of the notion of privacy if, in the future, a brain scan can reveal our deepest thoughts, feelings and intentions on a computer screen? Will such mind-reading evidence be admissible in the courtroom? Will it be used in interrogations of criminal suspects, of terrorists or of schoolchildren in the principal's office?

Kevin Warwick, Professor of Cybernetics at the University of Reading, had a device implanted in his arm that enabled his nervous system to communicate with a computer. In the future, implants into the retina or cochlea might permit enhanced vision or hearing, perhaps even seeing infrared frequencies or hearing ultrasound. Other examples of current research with ethical, legal and moral implications include the work of scientists who have taught monkeys, and more recently humans, to move cursors on computer screens by just thinking about or 'willing' it. The goal of this research is to make sophisticated brain–computer interface technologies that will improve the quality of life for people with disabilities or neurological diseases such as ALS (Chapin et al., 1999; Kennedy et al., 2000; Moore, 2003; Musallam et al., 2004). This, of course, is a noble goal, but the technology can also be used to enhance performance of the nondisabled as well.

The issue of enhancement, whether it is cosmetic surgery, gene manipulation or neural transplants, raises important ethical issues, such as the fairness with which the availability of the procedures will be provided, how to avoid coercion with regard to the use of the technology, and, to the extent that the enhancement might threaten human nature itself (for example, posthumanism), whether the technology should be pursued at all (Greely, 2006, p. 256). Will cognitive-enhancing drugs and genetic manipulation to improve academic or physical performance only be available to those people in a population who can afford to pay for it, or will a more equitable way of distributing these technologies be applied? Will a person have a choice in whether a 'mood-enhancing' drug is taken to increase workplace productivity, or will a worker be forced to take the drug or risk losing their job? What choice will or should children have if the enhancing technology is used during infancy or early childhood?

The discussion of neuroethics is in its infancy; however, many of the concerns over future technology coming from research in neuroscience and psychology have already been raised in the popular media. For example, the movie *Eternal Sunshine of the Spotless Mind* (2004) brings up the possibility of having unpleasant memories removed via stimulation to brain regions involved in memory storage. (What would replace these unwanted memories? They could be replaced by more pleasant 'virtual memories' such as sailing on the winner of the America's Cup, traveling to Tahiti, or knowledge of Spanish.) *Minority Report* is a movie released in 2002 about a future in which police use psychic technology to predict future criminal behavior and arrest the perpetrator before the actual crime can be committed. It just might turn out that the psychic technology of the future is actually brain scanning, which is able to image the brain during a lie or in the planning of a future criminal act. Current discussions in neuroethics concern, among other issues, whether the technologies coming from neuroscience research are leading to greater authoritarian control of our lives, and the extent to which 'profiling and prediction' on the basis of brain scans '... followed by the direct electromagnetic manipulation of neural processes or the targeted administration of drugs to "correct" or "normalize" undesirable profiles' is likely to be used in our future (Rose, 2005, p. 302). Certainly, as the subtitle of Steven Rose's book suggests, there are both promises and perils emerging in tomorrow's (and today's) neuroscience.

Searching for Truth

> I will go wherever the truth leads me … Lurie, if the Torah cannot go out into your world of scholarship and return stronger, then we are all fools and charlatans. I have faith in the Torah. I am not afraid of truth. (Potok, 1975, p. 391)

Chaim Potok's book *In the Beginning* (1975) is about a young Jewish man named David Lurie who starts to appreciate the value of scientific biblical criticism, but becomes very much aware of the problems and questions that sometimes develop when the understanding of scripture one once had is called into question by other apparently conflicting evidence. The quote above illustrates David's goal to pursue the truth, and the response given by his Rebbe/teacher that the Torah can stand up to any challenge coming from secular disciplines. The Rebbe charges David to continue seeking the truth, no matter where that truth might lead. We too can pursue the truth without fear of where that truth might take us, because as Christians we believe that all truth is God's truth. Because God is the author of all truth, the truth revealed in nature will not and cannot conflict with the truth revealed in scripture. Yes, our interpretation of what we read in nature using scientific methodology or in scripture using biblical scholarship might be in error (both scientists and biblical scholars or theologians are human), but the data of nature or of scripture cannot be contradictory if God is the author of both.

Research in neuroscience and psychology is increasingly shedding light on why we act, think and feel the way we do. The theory of evolution seems to be the best interpretation of the method God used to create. As Christians who are serious about the Bible but also aware of what science tells us about God's creation (including our own existence), it is important that we see the perspectives provided by science and religion as compatible and consistent, as 'going together'. John Habgood studied natural science and physiology at Cambridge University before pursuing his ordination in the Church of England, eventually becoming the Archbishop of York. He has written extensively on the relationship between science and religion, and the necessary unity (despite the apparent contradictions) between what is known through science and what is known through religious experience. In his book *Confessions of a Conservative Liberal* (1988), he makes the following observation:

> The word 'integrity' itself has two meanings. The first is 'honesty' … We have to be honest in facing our limitations, in facing the sheer complexity of the world, honest in facing criticism even of things which are deeply precious to us. But integrity also means wholeness, oneness, the desire for single vision, the refusal to split our minds into separate compartments where incompatible ideas are not allowed to come into contact … An undivided mind looks in the end for an undivided truth, a oneness at the heart of things. And this isn't just fantasy. The whole intellectual quest despite its fragmentation,

> despite its limitations and uncertainties, seems to presuppose that in the end we are all encountering a single reality, and single truth. (Habgood, 1988, p. 95)

As discussed in earlier chapters in this book, scientists sometimes go beyond their areas of expertise, or go beyond the legitimate boundaries of empirical science and make proclamations regarding topics that cannot be addressed using scientific methods. For example, we have all heard some scientist pontificate on the lack of meaning or purpose in the universe, a statement for which there is no empirical evidence, and a topic about which science cannot make any valid claim. Nevertheless, Christians can be confident that what is found and confirmed in neuroscientific and psychological research, when science as science and not as philosophy is practiced, will be complementary to what is learned through studying the Bible and through personal, religious experience. As Habgood indicates above, we are encountering a single reality, but that reality is a multileveled unity, and multiple perspectives are needed. Let us critically examine the findings of neuroscience and psychology as they relate to topics that touch on our religious faith. Let us make sure that the science (as well as the theology) is good. Let us also, however, be receptive to the findings that pass this kind of scrutiny, knowing with confidence that what is discovered at one level of reality, perhaps the biological level, is part of a larger picture which includes psychological, sociological and theological levels. This is God's world, and he tells us about it through many ways. Let us be ready to learn about this world (including learning about human beings) in all the ways God uses to communicate to us about what he has created.

Bibliography

Albright, C. R. (2000), 'The "God module" and the complexifying brain', *Zygon,* **35**, 735–44.

Allen, Robert and Scheidt, Stephen (1996), 'Empirical Basis for Cardiac Psychology', in Robert Allen and Stephen Scheidt (eds), *Heart & Mind: The Practice of Cardiac Psychology*, Washington, DC: American Psychological Association.

Amaral, David G. (2002), 'The primate amygdala and the neurobiology of social behavior: Implications for understanding social anxiety', *Biological Psychiatry*, **51**, 11–17.

Anderson, Steven W., Bechara, Antoine, Damasio, Hanna, Tranel, Daniel and Damasio, Antonio R. (1999), 'Impairment of social and moral behavior related to early damage in human prefrontal cortex', *Nature Neuroscience*, **2**, 1032–7.

Arehart-Treichel, Joan (2005), 'Clues to criminal mind found in prefrontal cortex', *Psychiatric News*, **40** (12), 22.

Armand, Nicholi M. Jr (2002), *The Question of God: C.S. Lewis and Sigmund Freud Debate God, Love, Sex, and the Meaning of Life*, New York: Free Press.

Ashbrook, James B. and Albright, Carol R. (1997), *The Humanizing Brain: Where Religion and Neuroscience Meet*, Cleveland, OH: Pilgrim Press.

Barber, Nigel (2004), *Kindness in a Cruel World: The Evolution of Altruism*, Amherst, NY: Prometheus Books.

Barbour, Ian G. (1966), *Issues in Science and Religion*, Englewood Cliffs, NJ: Prentice Hall.

Barbour, Ian G. (1990), *Religion in an Age of Science*, New York: HarperSanFrancisco.

Barbour, Ian G. (1997), *Religion and Science: Historical and Contemporary Issues*, New York: HarperSanFrancisco.

Barrett, Louise, Dunbar, Robin and Lycett, John (2002), *Human Evolutionary Psychology*, Princeton, NJ: Princeton University Press.

Barrow, John D. (2003), *The Constants of Nature: From Alpha to Omega – The Numbers that Encode the Deepest Secrets of the Universe*, New York: Pantheon Books.

Baumeister, Roy F., Smart, Laura and Boden, Joseph, M. (1996), 'Relation of threatened egotism to violence and aggression: The dark side of high self-esteem', *Psychological Review*, **103**, 5–33.

Beit-Hallahmi, Benjamin and Argyle, Michael (1997), *The Psychology of Religious Behaviour, Belief and Experience*, New York: Routledge.

Benson, Herbert, Dusek, Jeffery A., Sherwood, Jane B., Lam Peter, Bethea, Charles F., Carpenter, William, Levitsky, Sidney, Hill, Peter C., Clem, Donald W., Manoj, K. Jain, Drumel, David, Kopecky, Stephen L., Mueller, Paul S., Marek, Dean, Rollins, Sue and Hibberd, Patricia L. (2006), 'Study of the therapeutic effects of intercessory prayer (STEP) in cardiac bypass patients: A multicenter randomized trial of uncertainty and certainty of receiving intercessory prayer', *American Heart Journal*, **151**, 934–42.

Bhaskar, Roy (1997), *A Realist Theory of Science* (2nd edn), London: Verso.

Bhaskar, Roy (1998), *The Possibility of Naturalism* (3rd edn), London: Routledge.

Boyd, Craig A. (2004a), 'Thomistic Natural Law and the Limits of Evolutionary Psychology', in Philip Clayton and Jeffrey Schloss (eds), *Evolution and Ethics: Human Morality in Biological and Religious Perspective*, Grand Rapids, MI: Eerdmans.

Boyd, Craig A. (2004b), 'Was Thomas Aquinas a sociobiologist? Thomistic natural law, rational goods, and sociobiology', *Zygon*, **39**, 659–80.

Boyer, Pascal (2001), *Religion Explained: The Evolutionary Origins of Religious Thought*, New York: Basic Books.

Brooke, John Hedley (1991), *Science and Religion: Some Historical Perspectives*, Cambridge, UK: Cambridge University Press.

Brooke, John Hedley (2001). 'The Wilberforce–Huxley debate: Why did it happen?', *Science & Christian Belief*, **13**, 127–41.

Brown, Warren. S. (1998), 'Cognitive Contributions to Soul', in Warren S. Brown, Nancey Murphy and H. Newton Malony (eds), *Whatever Happened to the Soul? Scientific and Theological Portraits of Human Nature*, Minneapolis, MN: Fortress Press.

Brown, Warren. S., Murphy, Nancey and Malony, H. Newton (1998), *Whatever Happened to the Soul? Scientific and Theological Portraits of Human Nature*, Minneapolis, MN: Fortress Press.

Buller, David J. (2005), *Adapting Minds: Evolutionary Psychology and the Persistent Quest for Human Nature*, Cambridge, MA: MIT Press.

Buss, David M. (1995), 'Evolutionary psychology: A new paradigm for psychological science', *Psychological Inquiry*, **6**, 1–30.

Buss, David M. and Duntley, Joshua D. (2003), 'Homicide: An Evolutionary Psychological Perspective and Implications for Public Policy', in Richard W. Bloom and Nancy Dess (eds), *Evolutionary Psychology and Violence: A Primer for Policymakers and Public Policy Advocates*, Westport, CT: Praeger.

Buss, David M., Larsen, Randy J., Westen, Drew and Semmelroth, Jennifer (1992), 'Sex differences in jealousy: Evolution, physiology, and psychology', *Psychological Science*, **3**, 251–5.

Buunk, Bram P., Angleitner, Alois, Oubaid, Viktor and Buss, David M. (1996), 'Sex differences in jealousy in evolutionary and cultural perspective: Tests from the Netherlands, Germany, and the United States', *Psychological Science*, **7**, 359–63.

Byrd, Randolph C. (1988), 'Positive therapeutic effects of intercessory prayer in a coronary care unit population', *Southern Medical Journal*, **81**, 826–9.

Campbell, Heidi and Walker, Mark (2005), 'Religion and transhumanism: Introducing a conversation', *Journal of Evolution & Technology*, **14**, i–xiv.

Cardena, E., Lynn, S.J. and Krippner, S. (2000), *Varieties of Anomalous Experience*, Washington, DC: American Psychological Association.

Carlson, Neil R. (2007), *Physiology of Behavior* (9th edn), New York: Allyn and Bacon.

Chapin, John K., Moxon, Karen A., Markowitz, Ronald S. and Nicolelis, Miguel A.L. (1999), 'Real-time control of a robot arm using simultaneously recorded neurons in the motor cortex', *Nature Neuroscience*, **2**, 664–70.

Chu, J., Liston, B., Sieger, M. and Williams, D. (2004), 'Is God in our genes?', *Time*, **164**, 25 October, 62–72.

Coakley, Sarah (1997), 'Introduction: Religion and the Body', in Sarah Coakley (ed.), *Religion and the Body*, Cambridge: Cambridge University Press.

Collier, Andrew (1994), *Critical Realism: An Introduction to Roy Bhaskar's Philosophy*, London: Verso.

Commission on Children at Risk (2003), *Hardwired to Connect: The New Scientific Case for Authoritative Communities*, New York: Institute for American Values.

Cooper, John (2001), 'Biblical Anthropology and the Body–soul Problem', in Kevin Corcoran (ed.), *Soul Body and Survival: Essays on the Metaphysics of Human Persons*, Ithaca, NY: Cornell University Press.

Corcoran, Kevin (2001), *Soul, Body, and Survival: Essays on the Metaphysics of Human Persons*, Ithaca, NY: Cornell University Press.

Cummings, Jeffrey L. and Mega, Michael S. (2003), *Neuropsychiatry and Behavioral Neuroscience,* Oxford: Oxford University Press.

d'Aquili, Eugene G. and Newberg, Andrew B. (1999), *The Mystical Mind: Probing the Biology of Religious Experience*, Minneapolis, MN: Fortress Press.

Damasio, Antonio R. (1994), *Descartes' Error: Emotion, Reason, and the Human Brain*, New York: Avon.

Damasio, Antonio R. (1999), *The Feeling of What Happens: Body and Emotion in the Making of Consciousness*, New York: Harcourt Brace.

Darwin, Charles (1859/2003), *On the Origin of Species*, Cambridge, MA: Harvard University Press (original work published in 1859).

Davidson, Richard J. (2002), 'Anxiety and affective style: Role of prefrontal cortex and amygdala', *Biological Psychiatry*, **51**, 68–80.

Davidson, Richard J. and Irwin, William. (1999), 'The functional neuroanatomy of emotion and affective style', *Trends in Cognitive Sciences*, **3**, 11–21.

Davidson, Richard J., Jackson, Daren C. and Kalin, Ned H. (2000), 'Emotion, plasticity, context, and regulation: Perspectives from affective neuroscience', *Psychological Bulletin*, **126**, 890–909.

Dawkins, Richard (2003), *A Devil's Chaplain: Reflections on Hope, Lies, Science, and Love*, New York: Houghton Mifflin.

Dembski, William A. and Ruse, Michael (2004), *Debating Design: From Darwin to DNA*, Cambridge: Cambridge University Press.

Dhanani, Alnoor (2002), 'Islam', in Gary B. Ferngren (ed.), *Science & Religion: A Historical Introduction*, Baltimore, MD: Johns Hopkins Press.

Draper, John William (1874), *History of the Conflict between Religion and Science*, New York: D. Appleton.

Drees, Willem B. (1996), *Religion, Science and Naturalism*, New York: Cambridge.

Duntley, Joshua D. and Buss, David M. (2004), 'The Evolution of Evil', in Arthur G. Miller (ed.), *The Social Psychology of Good and Evil*, New York: Guilford Press.

Faber, M.D. (2004), *The Psychological Roots of Religious Belief*, Amherst, NY: Prometheus Books.

Farrow, Tom F.D., Zheng, Ying, Wilkinson, Iain D., Spence, Sean A., Deakin, J.F. William, Tarrier, Nick, Griffiths, Paul D. and Woodruff, Peter W.R. (2001), 'Investigating the functional anatomy of empathy and forgiveness', *NeuroReport*, **12**, 2433–8.

Feinberg, Todd E. (2001), *Altered Egos: How the Brain Creates the Self*, Oxford, UK: Oxford University Press.

Ferngren, Gary B. (2002), *Science & Religion: A Historical Introduction*, Baltimore, MD: Johns Hopkins University Press.

Finger, Stanley (1994), *Origins of Neuroscience: A History of Explorations into Brain Function*, Oxford: Oxford University Press.

Finger, Stanley (2000), *Minds behind the Brain: A History of the Pioneers and their Discoveries*, Oxford: Oxford University Press.

Fisher, Christopher L. (2005), 'Animals, humans and x-men: Human uniqueness and the meaning of personhood', *Theology and Science*, **3**, 291–314.

Gangestad, Steven W., Simpson, Jeffery A., Cousins, Alita J., Garver-Apgar, Christine E. and Christensen, P. Niels (2004), 'Women's preferences for male behavioral displays change across the menstrual cycle', *Psychological Science*, **15**, 203–7.

Gartner, John, Larson, Dave B. and Allen, George, D. (1991), 'Religious commitment and mental health: A review of the empirical literature', *Journal of Psychology and Theology*, **19**, 6–25.

Gaulin, Steven J.C. and McBurney, Donald H. (2004), *Evolutionary Psychology* (2nd edn), Upper Saddle River, NJ: Pearson.

Gay, Peter (1989), *The Freud Reader*, New York: W.W. Norton.

Giberson, Karl W. and Yerxa, Donald A. (2002), *Species of Origins: America's Search for a Creation Story*, New York: Rowman & Littlefield.

Goetz, Stewart (2005), 'Substance Dualism', in Joel B. Green and Stuart L. Palmer (eds), *In Search of the Soul: Four Views of the Mind-Body Problem*, Downers Grove, IL: InterVarsity Press.

Gould, Stephen Jay (2000), 'More Things in Heaven and Earth', in Hilary Rose and Steven Rose (eds), *Alas, Poor Darwin: Arguments Against Evolutionary Psychology*, New York: Harmony Books.

Grant, Edward (1996), *The Foundations of Modern Science in the Middle Ages: Their Religious, Institutional, and Intellectual Contexts*, Cambridge, UK: Cambridge University Press.

Greely, Henry T. (2006), 'The Social Effects of Advances in Neuroscience: Legal Problems, Legal Perspectives', in Judy Illes (ed.), *Neuroethics: Defining the Issues in Theory, Practice, and Policy*, Oxford, UK: Oxford University Press.

Green, Joel B. (2004a), *What About the Soul? Neuroscience and Christian Anthropology*, Nashville, TN: Abingdon Press.

Green, Joel B. (2004b), 'Resurrection of the Body: New Testament Voices Concerning Personal Continuity and the Afterlife', in Joel B. Green (ed.), *What About the Soul? Neuroscience and Christian Anthropology*, Nashville, TN: Abingdon Press.

Greene, Joshua D., Somerville, R. Brian, Nystrom, Leigth, E., Darley, John M. and Cohen, Jonathan D. (2001), 'An fMRI investigation of emotional engagement in moral judgment', *Science*, **293**, 2105–8.

Grinde, Bjorn (1998), 'The biology of religion: A Darwinian gospel', *Journal of Social & Evolutionary Systems*, **21**, 19–28.

Gutenson, Charles E. (2004), 'Time, Eternity, and Personal Identity: The Implications of Trinitarian Theology', in Joel B. Green (ed.), *What About the Soul? Neuroscience and Christian Anthropology,* Nashville, TN: Abingdon Press.

Habgood, John (1964), *Religion and Science*, London: Mills & Boon.

Habgood, John (1988), *Confessions of a Conservative Liberal*, London: SPCK.

Habgood, John (1998), *Being a Person: Where Faith and Science Meet*, London: Hodder & Stoughton.

Habgood, John (2002), *The Concept of Nature*, London: Darton, Longman & Todd.

Haidt, Jonathan (2001), 'The emotional dog and its rational tail: A social intuitionist approach to moral judgment', *Psychological Review*, **108**, 814–34.

Hamer, Dean (2004), *The God Gene: How Faith is Hardwired into our Genes*, New York: Doubleday.

Hardy, Alister (1966), *The Divine Flame: An Essay towards a Natural History of Religion*, Oxford: The Religious Experience Research Unit.

Harris, William S., Gowda, Manohar, Kolb, Jerry W., Strychacz, Christopher P., Vacek, James L., Jones, Phillip G., Forker, Alan, O'Keefe, James H., and McCallister, Ben D. (1999), 'A randomized, controlled trial of the effects of remote, intercessory prayer on outcomes in patients admitted to the coronary care unit', *Archives of Internal Medicine*, **159**, 2273–8.

Harrison, Peter (2006), '"Science" and "religion": Constructing the boundaries', *The Journal of Religion*, **86**, 81–106.

Haught, John F. (2000), *God after Darwin: A Theology of Evolution*, Boulder, CO: Westview Press.

Hay, David (1990), *Religious Experience Today: Studying the Facts*, London: Mowbray.

Hay, David (1994), '"The biology of God": What is the current status of Hardy's hypothesis?', *The International Journal for the Psychology of Religion*, **4**, 1–23.

Hay, David and Nye, Rebecca (1998), *The Spirit of the Child*, London: HarperCollins.

Hay, David and Socha, Pawel M. (2005), 'Spirituality as a natural phenomenon: Bringing biological and psychological perspectives together', *Zygon*, **40**, 589–612.

Heidelberger, Michael (2004), *Nature from Within: Gustav Theodor Fechner and his Psychophysical Worldview*, Pittsburgh, PA: University of Pittsburgh Press.

Heilman, Kenneth, M., Watson, Robert, T. and Valenstein, Edward (1993), 'Neglect and Related Disorders', in Kenneth M. Heilman and Edward Valenstein (eds), *Clinical Neuropsychology* (3rd edn), Oxford: Oxford University Press.

Hill, Peter C. and Butter, Eric. M. (1995), 'The role of religion in promoting physical health', *Journal of Psychology and Christianity*, **14**, 141–55.

Hill, Peter C. and Hood, Ralph W. Jr (1999), *Measures of Religiosity*, Birmingham, AL: Religious Education Press.

Hill, Peter C. and Pargament, Kenneth I. (2003), 'Advances in the conceptualization and measurement of religion and spirituality: Implications for physical and mental health research', *American Psychologist*, **58**, 64–74.

Jacobs, Lewis (1997), 'The Body in Jewish Worship: Three Rituals Examined', in Sarah Coakley (ed.), *Religion and the Body*, Cambridge, UK: Cambridge University Press.

James, William (1890/1950), *The Principles of Psychology*, New York: Dover (original work published 1890).

James, William (1902/1999), *The Varieties of Religious Experience*, New York: The Modern Library (original work published 1902).

Jeeves, Malcolm (2004a), *From Cells to Souls – and Beyond: Changing Portraits of Human Nature,* Grand Rapids, MI: Eerdmans.

Jeeves, Malcolm (2004b), 'Mind Reading and Soul Searching in the Twenty-First Century', in Joel B. Green (ed.), *What About the Soul?*, Nashville, TN: Abingdon Press.

Jones, Stanton (1994), 'A constructive relationship for religion with the science and profession of psychology: Perhaps the boldest model yet', *American Psychologist*, **49**, 184–99.

Joseph, R. (2001), 'The limbic system and the soul: Evolution and the neuroanatomy of religious experience', *Zygon*, **36**, 105–36.

Kennedy, P.R., Bakay, R.A.E., Moore, M.M., Adams, K. and Goldwaithe, J. (2000), 'Direct control of a computer from the human central nervous system', *IEEE Transactions on Rehabilitation Engineering*, **8**, 198–202.

Kiecolt-Glaser, Janice K., McGuire, Lynanne, Robles, Theodore F. and Glaser, Ronald (2002), 'Emotions, morbidity, and mortality: New perspectives from psychoneuroimmunology', *Annual Review of Psychology*, **53**, 83–107.

Kirkpatrick, Lee A. (2005), *Attachment, Evolution, and the Psychology of Religion*, New York: Guilford Press.

Knight, Robert G. (1992), *The Neuropsychology of Degenerative Brain Diseases*, Hillsdale, NJ: Lawrence Erlbaum.

Kober, Hedy, Ray, Alysa, Obhi, Sukhvinder, Guise, Kevin and Keenan, Julian Paul (2005), 'The Neural Correlates of Depersonalization: A Disorder of Self-Awareness', in Todd E. Feinberg and Julian Paul Keenan (eds), *The Lost Self: Pathologies of the Brain and Identity*, Oxford: Oxford University Press.

Koenig, Harold G. (1997), *Is Religion Good for your Health? The Effects of Religion on Physical and Mental Health*, New York: Haworth Pastoral Press.

Koenig, Harold G. (2002), 'The Connection between Psychoneuroimmunology and Religion', in Harold G. Koenig and Harvey Jay Cohen (eds), *The Link between Religion and Health: Psychoneuroimmunology and the Faith Factor,* Oxford: Oxford University Press.

Koenig, Harold G., McCullough, Michael E. and Larson, David B. (2001), *Handbook of Religion and Health*, Oxford: Oxford University Press.

Krantz, David S. and McCeney, Melissa K. (2002), 'Effects of psychological and social factors on organic disease: A critical assessment of research on coronary heart disease', *Annual Review of Psychology*, **53**, 341–69.

Krueger, Oliver (2005), 'Gnosis in cyberspace? Body, mind and progress in posthumanism', *Journal of Evolution & Technology*, **14**, 77–89.

Kuhn, Thomas S. (1970), *The Structure of Scientific Revolutions* (2nd edn), Chicago, IL: University of Chicago Press.

Kurzweil, Ray (2000), *The Age of Spiritual Machines: When Computers Exceed Human Intelligence*, New York: Penguin Books.

Kurzweil, Ray (2005), *The Singularity is Near: When Humans Transcend Biology*, New York: Viking.

La Mettrie, Julien Offray de (1748/1960), *L'homme Machine*, Princeton, NJ: Princeton University Press (original work published 1748).

Larson, Edward J. (1997), *Summer for the Gods: The Scopes Trial and America's Continuing Debate over Science and Religion*, Cambridge, MA: Harvard University Press.

Lazarus, Richard S. (1991), *Emotion & Adaptation*, New York: Oxford University Press.

Leahey, Thomas H. (1992), 'The mythical revolutions of American psychology', *American Psychologist*, **47**, 308–18.

Leahey, Thomas H. (2000), *A History of Psychology: Main Currents in Psychological Thought* (5th edn), Upper Saddle River, NJ: Prentice Hall.

Leahey, Thomas Hardy and Harris, Richard Jackson (2001), *Learning and Cognition* (5th edn), Upper Saddle River, NJ: Prentice Hall.

LeDoux, Joseph (1996), *The Emotional Brain*, New York: Touchstone.

Lee, Bruce. Y. and Newberg, Andrew B. (2005), 'Religion and health: A review and critical analysis', *Zygon*, **40**, 443–68.

Levin, Jeffrey S. and Chatters, Linda M. (1998), 'Research on Religion and Mental Health: An Overview of Empirical Findings and Theoretical Issues', in H.G. Koenig (ed.), *Handbook of Religion and Mental Health*, San Diego, CA: Academic Press.

Lindberg, David C. (2003), 'Galileo, the Church, and the Cosmos', in David C. Lindberg and Ronald L. Numbers (eds), *When Science & Christianity Meet*, Chicago, IL: University of Chicago Press.

Lindberg, David C. and Numbers, Ronald L. (1986), *God & Nature: Historical Essays on the Encounter between Christianity and Science*, Berkeley, CA: University of California Press.

Lindberg, David C. and Numbers, Ronald L. (2003), *When Science & Christianity Meet*, Chicago, IL: University of Chicago Press.

Looy, Heather (2004), 'Embodied and embedded morality: Divinity, identity, and disgust', *Zygon*, **39**, 219–35.

Looy, Heather (2005), 'The body of faith: Genetic and evolutionary considerations', *Journal of Psychology and Christianity*, **24**, 113–21.

Looy, Heather, Reimer, Kevin and Seybold, Kevin (2005), 'Reductive no more: Explaining religion without explaining it away', *Journal of Psychology and Christianity*, **24**, 101–4.

MacKay, Donald M. (1974), *The Clockwork Image: A Christian Perspective on Science*, Downers Grove, IL: InterVarsity Press.

Macmillan, Malcolm (2000), *An Odd Kind of Fame: Stories of Phineas Gage*, Cambridge, MA: MIT Press.

Marshall, Louise H. and Magoun, Horace, W. (1998), *Discoveries in the Human Brain: Neuroscience Prehistory, Brain Structure, and Function*, Totowa, NJ: Humana Press.

McGrath, Alister (1999), *Science and Religion: An Introduction*, Oxford: Blackwell.

McGrath, Alister (2001), *A Scientific Theology, Volume 1: Nature*, Grand Rapids, MI: Eerdmans.

McGrath, Alister (2002), *A Scientific Theology, Volume 2: Reality*, Grand Rapids, MI: Eerdmans.

McGrath, Alister (2003), *A Scientific Theology, Volume 3: Theory*, Grand Rapids, MI: Eerdmans.

McGrath, Alister (2004a), *The Twilight of Atheism*, New York: Doubleday.

McGrath, Alister (2004b), *The Science of God: An Introduction to Scientific Theology*, London: T&T Clark International.

McGrath, Alister (2005), *Dawkins' God: Genes, Memes, and the Meaning of Life*, Oxford: Blackwell.

McNamara, Patrick (2001), 'Religion and the Frontal Lobes', in Jensine Andresen (ed.), *Religion in Mind*, New York: Cambridge University Press.

McNamara, Patrick (2002), 'The motivational origins of religious practices', *Zygon*, **37**, 143–60.

Mesulam, M.-M. (2000), 'Attentional Networks, Confusional States and Neglect Syndromes', in M.-M. Mesulam (ed.), *Principles of Behavioral and Cognitive Neurology*, Oxford: Oxford University Press.

Midgley, Mary (2002), *Evolution as a Religion*, New York: Routledge.

Miller, Kenneth R. (1999), *Finding Darwin's God: A Scientist's Search for Common Ground between God and Evolution*, New York: Harper Perennial.

Miller, Todd Q., Smith, Timothy W., Turner, Charles W., Guijarro, Margarita L. and Hallet, Amanda J. (1996), 'A meta analytic review of research on hostility and physical health', *Psychological Bulletin*, **119**, 322–48.

Moll, Jorge, de Oliveira-Souza, Ricardo, Eslinger, Paul J., Bramati, Ivanei E., Mourão-Miranda, Janaína, Andreiuolo, Pedro A. and Pessoa, Luiz (2002), 'The neural correlates of moral sensitivity: A functional magnetic resonance imaging investigation of basic and moral emotions', *The Journal of Neuroscience*, **22**, 2730–36.

Moore, Melody M. (2003), 'Real-world applications for brain-computer interface technology', *IEEE Transactions on Neural Systems and Rehabilitation Engineering*, **11**, 162–5.

Moravec, Hans (1988), *Mind Children: The Future of Robot and Human Intelligence*, Cambridge, MA: Harvard University Press.

Moravec, Hans (1999), *Robot: Mere Machines to Transcendent Mind*, Oxford: Oxford University Press.

Morris, Simon Conway (2003), *Life's Solution: Inevitable Humans in a Lonely Universe*, Cambridge: Cambridge University Press.

Murphy, Nancey (2005), 'Nonreductive Physicalism', in Joel B. Green and Stuart L. Palmer (eds), *In Search of the Soul: Four Views of the Mind-Body Problem*, Downers Grove, IL: InterVarsity Press.

Murphy, Nancey (2006), *Bodies and Souls, or Spirited Bodies?*, Cambridge, UK: Cambridge University Press.

Musallam, S., Corneil, B.D., Greger, B., Scherberger, H. and Andersen, R.A. (2004), 'Cognitive control signals for neural prosthetics', *Science*, **305**, 258–62.

Myers, David G. (2005), *Exploring Psychology* (6th edn), New York: Worth.

Newberg, Andrew and d'Aquili, Eugene (2001), *Why God Won't Go Away: Brain Science and the Biology of Belief*, New York: Ballantine Books.

Newberg, Andrew B., d'Aquili, Eugene G., Newberg, Stephanie K. and deMarici, Verushka (2000), 'The Neuropsychological Correlates of Forgiveness', in Michael E. McCullough, Kenneth I. Pargament and Carl E. Thoresen (eds), *Forgiveness: Theory, Research, and Practice*, New York: Guilford Press.

Numbers, Ronald L. (2006), *The Creationists: From Scientific Creationism to Intelligent Design*, Cambridge: HarvardUniversity Press.

O'Craven, K.M. and Kanwisher, N. (2000), 'Mental imagery of faces and places activates corresponding stimulus-specific brain regions', *Journal of Cognitive Neuroscience*, **12**, 1013–23.

Palmer, Stuart L. (2005), 'Christian Life and Theories of Human Nature', in Joel B. Green and Stuart L. Palmer (eds), *In Search of the Soul: Four Views of the Mind-Body Problem*, Downers Grove, IL: InterVarsity Press.

Pargament, Kenneth. I. (1997), *The Psychology of Religion and Coping*, New York: Guilford Press.

Pennock, Robert T. (2001), *Intelligent Design Creationism and its Critics: Philosophical, Theological, and Scientific Perspectives*, Cambridge, MA: MIT.

Persinger, Michael A. (1987), *Neuropsychological Bases of God Beliefs*, New York: Praeger.

Persinger, Michael A. (2002), 'Experimental Simulation of the God Experience: Implications for Religious Beliefs and the Future of the Human Species', in R. Joseph (ed.), *NeuroTheology: Brain, Science, Spirituality, Religious Experience*, San Jose, CA: University Press, California.

Peters, Ted (1999), 'Resurrection of the Very Embodied Soul?', in Robert John Russell, Nancey Murphy, Theo C. Meyering and Michael A. Arbib (eds), *Neuroscience and the Person: Scientific Perspectives on Divine Action*, Vatican City: Vatican Observatory Foundation.

Pickren, Wade E. (2000), 'A whisper of salvation: American psychologists and religion in the popular press, 1884–1908', *American Psychologist*, **55**, 1022–4.

Polanyi, Michael (1958), *Personal Knowledge: Towards a Post-critical Philosophy*, Chicago, IL: University of Chicago Press.

Popper, Karl R. and Eccles, John C. (1981), *The Self and its Brain*, New York: Springer International.

Port, Richard L. and Seybold, Kevin. S. (1995), 'Hippocampal synaptic plasticity as a biological substrate underlying episodic psychosis', *Biological Psychiatry*, **37**, 318–24.

Port, Richard L., Sample, John A. and Seybold, Kevin S. (1991), 'Partial hippocampal pyramidal cell loss alters behavior in rats: Implications for an animal model of schizophrenia', *Brain Research Bulletin*, **26**, 993–6.

Potok, Chaim (1975), *In the Beginning*, New York: Knopf.

Powell, Lynda H., Shahabi, Leila and Thoresen, Carl E. (2003), 'Religion and spirituality: Linkages to physical health', *American Psychologist*, **58**, 36–52.

Putnam, Robert D. (2000), *Bowling Alone: The Collapse and Revival of American Community*, New York: Simon & Schuster.

Pyysiäinen, Ilkka (2001), 'Cognition, Emotion, and Religious Experience', in Jensine Andresen (ed.), *Religion in Mind*, New York: Cambridge University Press.

Ramachandran, V.S. and Blakeslee, Sandra (1998), *Phantoms in the Brain: Probing the Mysteries of the Human Mind*, New York: Quill.

Ramírez-Johnson, Johnny, Fayard, Carlos, Garberoglio, Carlos and Ramírez, Clara M. Jorge (2002), 'Is faith an emotion? Faith as a meaning-making affective process: An example from breast cancer patients', *American Behavioral Scientist*, **45**, 1839–53.

Rizzolatti, Giacomo and Craighero, Laila (2004), 'The mirror-neuron system', *Annual Review of Neuroscience*, **27**, 169–92.

Rose, Steven (2005), *The Future of the Brain: The Promise and Perils of Tomorrow's Neuroscience*, Oxford: Oxford University Press.

Sacks, Oliver (1995), *An Anthropologist on Mars*, New York: Alfred A. Knopf.

Sacks, Oliver (1998), *The Man Who Mistook His Wife for a Hat*, New York: Touchstone.

Salovey, Peter, Rothman, Alexander, J., Detweiler, Jerusha B. and Steward, Wayne T. (2000), 'Emotional states and physical health', *American Psychologist*, **55**, 110–21.

Sanders, John (1998), *The God who Risks: A Theology of Providence*, Downers Grove, IL: InterVarsity Press.

Schloss, Jeffrey P. (2004). 'Evolutionary Ethics and Christian Morality: Surveying the Issues', in Philip Clayton and Jeffrey Schloss (eds), *Evolution and Ethics: Human Morality in Biological and Religious Perspective*, Grand Rapids, MI: Eerdmans.

Seeman, Teresa E., Dubin, Linda F. and Seeman, Melvin (2003), 'Religiosity/spirituality and health: A critical review of the evidence for biological pathways', *American Psychologist*, **58**, 53–63.

Sethi, Shenna and Seligman, Martin E.P. (1993), 'Optimism and fundamentalism', *Psychological Science*, **4**, 256–9.

Seybold, Kevin S. (2005), 'The untidiness of integration: John Stapylton Habgood', *Perspectives on Science and Christian Faith*, **57**, 114–19.

Seybold, Kevin S. and Hill, Peter C. (2001), 'The role of religion and spirituality in mental and physical health', *Current Directions in Psychological Science*, **10**, 21–4.

Seybold, Kevin S., Hill, Peter C., Neumann, Joseph K. and Chi, David S. (2001), 'Physiological and psychological correlates of forgiveness', *Journal of Psychology and Christianity*, **20**, 264–73.

Shults, F. LeRon (1999), *The Postfoundationalist Task of Theology: Wolfhart Pannenberg and the New Theological Rationality*, Grand Rapids, MI: Eerdmans.

Shults, F. LeRon (2003), *Reforming Theological Anthropology: After the Philosophical Turn to Relationality*, Grand Rapids, MI: Eerdmans.

Shults, R. LeRon (2005), *Reforming the Doctrine of God*, Grand Rapids, MI: Eerdmans.

Skinner, B.F. (1953), *Science and Human Behavior*, New York: The Free Press.

Skinner, B.F. (1976), *Walden Two*, New York: Macmillan.

Spilka, Bernard, Hood, Ralph W. Jr, Hunsberger, Bruce and Gorsuch, Richard (2003), *The Psychology of Religion: An Empirical Approach* (3rd edn), New York: Guilford Press.

Staune, Jean (2005), 'Darwinism design and purpose: A European perspective', paper presented at Metanexus Institute conference 'Science and Religion: Global Perspectives' 4–8 June, Philadelphia, PA.

Stone, Lawson G. (2004), 'The Soul: Possession, Part, or Person? The Genesis of Human Nature in Genesis 2:7', in Joel B. Green (ed.), *What About the Soul? Neuroscience and Christian Anthropology*, Nashville, TN: Abingdon Press.

Thoresen, Carl E. (1999), 'Spirituality and health: Is there a relationship?', *Journal of Health Psychology*, **4**, 291–300.

Thoresen, Carl E., Harris, Alex H.S. and Luskin, Frederic. (2000), 'Forgiveness and Health: An Unanswered Question', in Michael E. McCullough, Kenneth I. Pargament and Carl E. Thoresen (eds), *Forgiveness: Theory, Research, and Practice*, New York: Guilford Press.

Thoresen, Carl E., Harris, Alex H.S. and Oman, Doug (2001), 'Spirituality, Religion, and Health: Evidence, Issues, and Concerns', in Thomas G. Plante and Allen C. Sherman (eds), *Faith and Health: Psychological Perspectives*, New York: Guilford Press.

Thornhill, Randy and Palmer, Craig T. (2000), *A Natural History of Rape: Biological Bases of Sexual Coercion*, Cambridge, MA: MIT.

Uchino, Bert N., Uno, Darcy and Holt-Lunstad, Julianne (1999), 'Social support, physiological processes, and health', *Current Directions in Psychological Science*, **8**, 145–8.

Van Biema, David (compiler) (2005), 'Can You Believe in God and Evolution?', *Time*, **166**, 15 August, 34–5.

Van Leeuwen, Mary Stewart (2001), 'Of hoggamus and hogwash: Evolutionary psychology and gender relations', *Journal of Psychology and Theology*, **30**, 101–11.

Van Till, Howard J. (2001), 'The Creation: Intelligently Designed or Optimally Equipped?', in Robert T. Pennock (ed.), *Intelligent Design Creationism and its Critics: Philosophical, Theological, and Scientific Perspectives*, Cambridge, MA: MIT Press.

Vitz, Paul C. (1977), *Psychology as Religion: The Cult of Self-worship*, Grand Rapids, MI: Eerdmans.

Vogeley, Kai, Kurthen, Martin, Falkai, Peter and Maier, Wolfgang (1999), 'Essential functions of the human self model are implemented in the prefrontal cortex', *Consciousness and Cognition*, **8**, 343–63.

Waller, Niels G., Kojetin, Brian A., Bouchard, Thomas J. Jr, Lykken, David T. and Tellegen, Auke (1990), 'Genetic and environmental influences on religious interests, attitudes, and values: A study of twins reared apart and together', *Psychological Science*, **1**, 138–42.

Ward, Keith (2004), *The Case for Religion*, Oxford: Oneworld.

Ware, Kallistos (1997), 'My Helper and My Enemy': The Body in Greek Christianity', in Sarah Coakley (ed.), *Religion and the Body*, Cambridge: Cambridge University Press.

Warwick, Kevin (2000, February), 'Cyborg 1.0', *Wired Magazine*, **8.02**.

Waters, Brent (2006), *From Human to Posthuman: Christian Theology and Technology in a Postmodern World*, Aldershot: Ashgate.

Watson, John D. (1913), 'Psychology as the behaviorist views it', *Psychological Review*, **20**, 158–77.

Watters, Wendell (1992), *Deadly Doctrine: Health, Illness, and Christian God-talk*, Amherst, NY: Prometheus Books.

Watts, Fraser N. (1997), 'Psychological and religious perspectives on emotion', *Zygon*, **32**, 243–60.

Weaver, Glenn (2004), 'Embodied Spirituality: Experiences of Identity and Spiritual Suffering among Persons with Alzheimer's Dementia', in Malcolm Jeeves (ed.), *From Cells to Souls – and Beyond: Changing Portraits of Human Nature*, Grand Rapids, MI: Eerdmans.

White, Andrew Dickson (1896), *A History of the Warfare of Science with Theology in Christendom*, New York: D. Appleton.

Will, George (2005), 'Have a nice day, or else', *The Washington Post*, 21 April, p. A23.

Williams, J.H.G., Whiten, A., Suddendorf, T. and Perrett, D.I. (2001), 'Imitation, mirror neurons and autism', *Neuroscience and Biobehavioral Reviews*, **25**, 287–95.

Williams, Patricia A. (2001), *Doing without Adam and Eve: Sociobiology and Original Sin*, Minneapolis, MN: Fortress Press.

Wilson, David Sloan (2002), *Darwin's Cathedral: Evolution, Religion, and the Nature of Society*, Chicago, IL: University of Chicago Press.

Wilson, Edward O. (1998), *Concilience: The Unity of Knowledge*, New York: Vintage.

Witvliet, Charlotte van Oyen, Ludwig, Thomas E. and Vander Laan, Kelly L. (2001), 'Granting forgiveness or harboring grudges: Implications for emotion, physiology, and health', *Psychological Science*, **12**, 117–23.

Wolford, George, Miller, Michael B. and Gazzaniga, Michael (2000), 'The left hemisphere's role in hypothesis formation', *The Journal of Neuroscience*, **20**, RC 64–7.

Worthington, Everett L. (1998), 'The Pyramid Model of Forgiveness: Some Interdisciplinary Speculations about Unforgiveness and the Promotion of Forgiveness', in Everett L. Worthington (ed.), *Dimensions of Forgiveness: Psychological Research,* Philadelphia, PA: Templeton Foundation Press.

Worthington, Everett L. (2001), 'Unforgiveness, Forgiveness, and Reconciliation and their Implications for Societal Interventions', in Raymond G. Helmick and

Rodney L. Petersen (eds), *Forgiveness and Reconciliation: Religion, Public Policy, and Conflict Transformation*, Philadelphia, PA: Templeton Foundation Press.

Worthington, Everett L., Berry, Jack W. and Parrott, Les (2001), 'Unforgiveness, Forgiveness, Religion, and Health', in Thomas G. Plante and Allen C. Sherman (eds), *Faith and Health: Psychological Perspectives*, New York: Guilford Press.

Zimmer, Carl (2004), *Soul Made Flesh: The Discovery of the Brain – and How it Changed the World*, New York: Free Press.

Index